SOCIAL DETERMINANTS, HEALTH EQUITY AND HUMAN DEVELOPMENT

EDITOR

Boutayeb A.

Department of Mathematics Faculty of Sciences, Boulevard Mohamed VI, Oujda, Morocco.

CONTENT

SOCIAL DETERMINANTS, HEALTH EQUITY AND HUMAN DEVELOPMENT

FOREWORD

Satellite television has for many years brought to the attention of the world, the plight of the citizens of lessdeveloped countries who do not have the benefits of a good quality healthcare system. There is a distinction to be made between rich countries that do not provide a state-run system for their poorer citizens and those countries that cannot provide such care because their economies are not sufficiently strong to meet the costs involved. The book concentrates on the latter, and the contributors highlight the widening gap between the quality of healthcare services available in poor and rich countries.

In the recent past, improving the quality of healthcare was invariably a low priority for policy makers in developing countries where, additionally, government expenditure often benefitted a country's richest people more than its poorest, in absolute terms. In the second half of the last century, for which data are available, achievements in human development worldwide were uneven and were characterized by significant regional variations within less-developed countries. Large numbers of poor people in remote regions still have to travel huge distances to reach the nearest health facility, and then face lengthy delays in long queues to see a doctor or nurse. This contrasts sharply with urban populations, including those in poorer countries. These observations apply especially to the Continents of Africa, Oceania, South America and Asia, all of which have less-developed countries within their borders.

In the developed world dramatic changes are occurring in the delivery of healthcare. These changes are driven by economic factors, political and consumer will, ageing populations, demographic spreads, improved healthcare methods, and greater expectations. In the less-developed world, change is much slower but there are signs in some of these countries that the development of technology to support tele-medicine and e-health systems is quickening, thanks to the provision of data communication systems and mobile telephone networks. These have aided significantly the overworked key staff in the health services. There is a need to provide key aid workers, including paramedics, to health services in developing countries who have the necessary blend of technical skills and managerial flair to initiate and manage the introduction of (donated) new technologies. The introduction of computer networks worldwide will enable the governments of lessdeveloped countries to provide a greater level of service nearer to the patient, by setting-up electronic links to consultants many hundreds of kilometres away in regional hubs.

The contributors to this book have, collectively, many years' experience of charting, observing, measuring, analysing, and predicting the outcomes of the provision of healthcare in North Africa, particularly Morocco, and, in their contributions, they show a thorough understanding of the Continent's needs. It is to be hoped that, in the coming decades, governments will be able to provide what is needed to stave off the likely disasters associated with poor healthcare and other avoidable health-related factors that have a bearing on a nation's prosperity. Governments of countries on other continents may wish to heed the warnings and predictions reported in this book, for they have a significant bearing on the future and well-being of their people, too.

E.H. Twizell
Professor Emeritus
Brunel University, UK

PREFACE

The year 2008 marked the celebration of three important events related to health: the 60th anniversary of the creation of the World Health Organization, the 60th anniversary of the Human Right Declaration and the 30th anniversary of the Declaration of Alma Ata on primary health care. These three anniversaries coincide with the renewal hope in public health to reach the goal of "Health for All". Worldwide, many voices were raised to stress that the gap in access to health services is becoming wider and wider instead of narrowing. Today more than ever, the call is for justice in health between and within countries. The WHO Report 2008 and the declaration released by the WHO Commission on Social Determinants of Health are just two sources amongst many others dealing with social inequalities and equity in health, stressing that health is a human right and not a private commodity.

Studies in developed and developing countries have shown that the poor suffer more from high rates of illness than the rich. Lack of food, poor housing, unclean water, inappropriate sanitation, environment degradation, unsafe sex and difficult access to health services and health personnel are all behind infectious diseases and malnutrition. Overweight, smoking, alcohol, hypertension, and physical inactivity are the major risks linked to non-communicable diseases.

Although the last decade has seen a growing interest in the disease burden and how to reduce it, many strategies like those of the Millennium Development Goals remain based on global indicators representing average national numbers, often hiding inadmissible inequalities and disparities.

The nine chapters of this book have a common denominator, which is social determinant of health, equity and human development. The first chapter deals with measurements and indicators. It gives some definitions and concepts illustrated with concrete examples. The emphasis is on the necessity of equity analysis going beyond average numbers. The second chapter illustrates the link between social determinants, health equity and development through the health risks lenses. The third chapter is a review of selected recent references on equity and social determinants. The fourth chapter is devoted to the relation between equity and the disease burden. The fifth and sixth chapters consider respectively the case of obesity-diabetes and the Dengue disease. Chapter seven analyses inequalities and disparities in North Africa. Chapter eight is a commentary on fifty years of development in Morocco, stressing the necessity of equity analysis. Finally, chapter nine gives an overview of conventions and declarations adopted on children's rights, compared with the real situation of children in the world and illustrated by a case study of Gaza's children.

We hope that this humble book will contribute to the efforts endeavouring to establish more justice in access to health by understanding and acting on the relation between social determinants, health equity and human development.

Boutayeb Abdesslam
University Mohamed Ier
Morocco

CONTRIBUTORS

Aguenaou H.

Unité Mixte de Recherche en Nutrition et Alimentation, University Ibn Tofail, Kenitra-CNESTEN-Rabat, Morocco.

Bensouda Y.

Institut National d'Oncologie Service Oncologie Médicale, Rabat, Morocco.

Boutayeb A.

Department of Mathematics Faculty of Sciences, Boulevard Mohamed VI, Oujda, Morocco.

Boutayeb S.

Institut National d'Oncologie Service Oncologie Médicale, Rabat, Morocco.

Derouich M.

Department of Mathematics Faculty of Sciences, Boulevard Mohamed VI, Oujda, Morocco

Mehdad S.

Unité Mixte de Recherche en Nutrition et Alimentation, University Ibn Tofail, Kenitra-CNESTEN-Rabat, Morocco

Mokhtar N.

Unité Mixte de Recherche en Nutrition et Alimentation, University Ibn Tofail, Kenitra-CNESTEN-Rabat, Morocco

CHAPTER 1

Measurements and Indicators: Definitions, Concepts and Examples

Abdesslam Boutayeb[1,*] and Saber Boutayeb[2]

[1]*Department of Mathematics Faculty of Sciences, Boulevard Mohamed VI, BP: 717 Oujda, Morocco;
Email: x.boutayeb@menara.ma*

[2]*Institut National d'Oncologie Service Oncologie Médicale, Rabat, Morocco;
Email: boutayebdr@yahoo.fr*

Abstract: The importance of equity in health necessitates concise definitions of concepts and tools used either to describe the distribution of ill-health as a phenomenon in time and space, or to understand the causes underlying unfair and avoidable inequalities in order to act on them. Consequently, the measures of health inequalities depend on the approach adopted to distinguish different groups of a population (by sex, socioeconomic status, education level, residence area, income, ethnic groups, ...), the health variable to be described (mortality, morbidity, expectancy, quality of life, nutrition, access to services, ...), and the methods and tools for description and analysis (absolute numbers, relative differences, odd ratios, concentration index, regression, component analysis, discriminant analysis, ...). This first chapter is dedicated to the main concepts and indicators related to health measurements. Illustrative examples are given and clarifications are provided through remarks and discussions.

Keywords: Measurements, indicators, communicable diseases, human development, mortality, cost-benefit.

1. INTRODUCTION

The importance of equity in health necessitates concise definitions of concepts and tools used either to describe the distribution of ill-health as a phenomenon in time and space, or to understand the causes underlying unfair and avoidable inequalities in order to act on them. Consequently, the measures of health inequalities depend on the approach adopted to distinguish different groups of a population (by sex, socioeconomic status, education level, residence area, income, ethnic groups, ...), the health variable to be described (mortality, morbidity, expectancy, quality of life, nutrition, access to services, ...), and the methods and tools for description and analysis (absolute numbers, relative differences, odd ratios, concentration index, regression, component analysis, discriminant analysis, ...). This first chapter is a preamble to the remaining chapters of the book. It introduces the reader to different concepts and indictors related to health. Illustrative examples are given in each case, followed by remarks and discussions clarifying situations that may appear ambiguous. The main message is to attract attention on the understanding of average numbers usually largely used by decision makers and media to describe Gross Domestic Product, Human Development Index, Millennium Development Goals, Life Expectancy, Mortality Rate and other indicators. These average numbers often hide important and inadmissible inequalities and disparities. The examples discussed in this chapter show clearly the need to go beyond goals fixed in terms of average numbers, by looking also and more deeply at the crucial problem of unfair and avoidable inequalities.

2. STATISTICAL VALUES

2.1 Concepts and Definitions

In epidemiology and statistics in general, crude numbers are very often transformed and replaced by single values summarizing the whole set of data. Two main classes of statistical values are used. The first class comprises values indicating the general trend (also called measures of location), measured generally by the mean (average), median, midpoint and mode (the most frequent non missing value). The mean being the most used in this set.

The second class comprises measurements of variation. It completes the information of the first class by indicating how the observations are scattered or distributed around their mean. The commonly used statistics in this group are the variance, standard deviation (square root of variance), the range (span between the minimum and maximum values) and quintiles. The standard deviation is the most used.

---

*Corresponding author

2.2 Remark

As we will see in the next sections, health indicators measuring maternal mortality, infant mortality, access to antenatal and postnatal care and health status in general are given in the form of averages like those fixed in the Millennium Development Goals for example. Such considerations may be misleading when strategies are evaluated. Indeed, a country may improve globally a certain indicator (infant mortality for instance) by improving maternal health of urban populations (or rich and middle class) and exacerbating the dire conditions of rural populations (or lowest socioeconomic class). In this case, the indicator is improved in average but inequity is persistent or even accentuated.

2.3 Examples

2.3.1 Example1. Gross Domestic Product

The national income of a country is often measured by the Gross Domestic Product (GDP). The GDP can be quantified by the following formula:

GDP = consumption + gross investment + government expenditure + (exports – imports). Slightly different, the Gross National Product (GNP) uses net foreign income instead of net exports and imports. In other words, GDP is the total output produced in country in one year and expressed in market value. One of the most used indicators for economic comparison between countries is GDP *per capita*, obtained by dividing the country's GDP by the total population of the country. In other words, GDP per capita can be considered as a proxy of the value of goods produced per person in a given country. It is often expressed in purchasing power parity (PPP) (international US dollar). Ideally efficient markets, identical goods should have only one price. According to the World Bank, countries are worldwide classified into three groups. High income (GDP *per capita* > **US\$9,205**), Upper-middle income (GDP *per capita* **US\$2,976- US\$9,205**), Lower-middle income (GDP *per capita* **US\$745- US\$2,976**) and Low income (GDP *per capita* **<US\$745**)

For the year 2007, estimates of the Gross Domestic Product per capita are given by The World Bank for most countries of the world [1]. The world average GDP *per capita* was estimated at US\$ 8,219. In fact this is an artificial (theoretical) value obtained by assuming that the global world GDP is equally shared by all countries and all people around the world. Unfortunately, the share of resources is far from being equitable. Indeed, if we look at the GDP *per capita* of different countries, we are struck by the spectre of income: Burundi(115), Bangladesh(427), Benin(601), Pakistan(884), India(1,042) Angola(3,440), Argentina(6,641), France(41,523), Denmark(56,271), Iceland(62,733) and Luxembourg(99,879). The range, expressed as the gap between the lowest and the highest GDP is (99,879- 115=99,764), just unbelievable!

2.3.2 Example2. Human Development Index (HDI)

A comparison between countries based on increase in national income alone does not capture development in its fullest sense. Human development of nations goes beyond their economic wealth. To this end, five main composite indices were developed by the United Nations to measure the average achievements in basic human development (human development index (HDI), gender-related development index (GDI), human poverty indices (HPI-1 and HPI-2) and the gender empowerment measure (GEM) [2]. HDI is the most used index giving a summary measure of human development and allowing for a yearly comparison between countries around the world (Table **1**) and indicating the relative ranking evolution in time of each country (Table **2**)[2-4]. HDI is a three dimensional composite index obtained as a mean of three indicators weighed equally: health (life expectancy at birth), standard of living (GDP per capita) and education (literacy and enrolment) (see box).

Box

In general, to transform a raw variable X, into a unit-free indicator between 0 and 1, the following formula is used:

x-index = (X-minX)/(maxX-minX)

where minX and maxX are respectively the minimum an maximum that can be reached by the variable X.

The Human Development Index (HDI) then represents the average of the following three general indices:

Life Expectancy Index=(LE-25)/(85-25)

Adult Literacy Index=(AL-0)/(100-0)

Gross Enrollment Index=(GE-0)/(100-0)

Education Index = (2/3)ALI+(1/3)GEI

GDP Index= (log(GDP per capita)- log(100))/(log(40000)-log(100)

HDI = (1/3)[LEI+EI+GDPI]

End box

2.3.3 Remark

Countries are classed into three groups according to their level of human development. Countries with a HDI at least 0.800 belong to the highest development group, those with HDI at least 0.500 but less than 0.800 are said to have medium development, and finally the low development group comprises the least developed countries with HDI less than 0.500.

According to the United Nation Development Programme (UNDP) estimates released in December 2008, the average world HDI was: 0.747. But, worldwide, human development is uneven. The index varies from 0.968 for the highest development to 0.329 for the lowest development (see Table **1**).

Table 1. Classification of countries by HDI as published by UNDP in December 2008

High development (DHI >0.800)	Medium development (0.500 <HDI <0.800)	Low development HDI <0.5000
1 Iceland (0.968)	76 Turkey (0.798)	154 Nigeria (0.499)
2 Norway (0.968)	77 Dominica (0.797)	155 Lesotho (0.496)
3 Canada (0.967)	78 Lebanon (0.796)	156 Uganda (0.493)
4 Australia (0.965)	79 Peru (0.988)	157 Angola (0.484)
5 Ireland (0.960)	80 Colombia (0787)	158 Timor-Leste (0.483)
.	.	.
.	.	.
.	.	.
71 Kazakhstan (0.807)	149 Pap N Guinea (0.516)	175. Mozambique (0.366)
72 Ecuador (0.807)	150 Cameroon (0.514)	176 Liberia (0.364)
73 Russia (0.806)	151 Djibouti (05.513)	177. Dem Rep Congo (0.361)
74. Mauritius (0.802)	152 Thailand (0503)	178. Centre Africa (0.352)
75 Bosnia & Herz (0.802)	153 Senegal(0.502)	179 Sierra Leone (0.329)

3. MORTALITY AND MORBIDITY

3.1 Disease Classification (As Defined in WHO Reports)

3.1.1 Groups of Diseases

The World Health Organization classifies deaths using a tree structure. Three broad cause Groups are considered:

Group I: Communicable, maternal, prenatal and nutritional conditions

Group II: non communicable diseases (or chronic)

Group III: Injuries

Then each group is subdivided into sub-categories which in turn are again subdivided.

3.1.2 Remark

The terms chronic and non communicable are often used interchangeably because they are both related to incurable diseases of long periods. On the other hand, the term communicable is usually used for infectious diseases that are biologically transmitted either from human to human (measles, HIV, tuberculosis...) or through vectors (malaria, dengue, sleeping sickness,...). It is not so easy, however, to draw a line separating chronic diseases from communicable diseases. Several studies are being devoted to the frontier between these two classes of illnesses.

In the era of globalisation and information communication, although diseases like cancer, diabetes and cardiovascular diseases are not infectious, they are generally associated with risk factors that are highly communicated from one population to another. Smoking, alcohol, fast foods and inactivity are illustrative examples cross countries.

Evidence is linking a growing number of infectious agents to an increased risk of cancer.

According to the International Agency for Research on Cancer (IARC), cancers attributable to an infectious agent are thought to account for 26% of all cancers in developing countries and 8% of all cancers in the industrialised world.

Infections with several viruses, bacteria, and parasites increase the risk of human cancers of the cervix, liver, urinary bladder, and stomach and can also cause leukaemia. There is also increasing evidence that influenza can trigger coronary and vascular events.

3.1.3 Example

As shown by the figure below, deaths caused by non communicable diseases dominate the mortality statistics in five out of six regions of the World Health Organization [3]. The exception is Africa where deaths caused by communicable diseases are predominant.

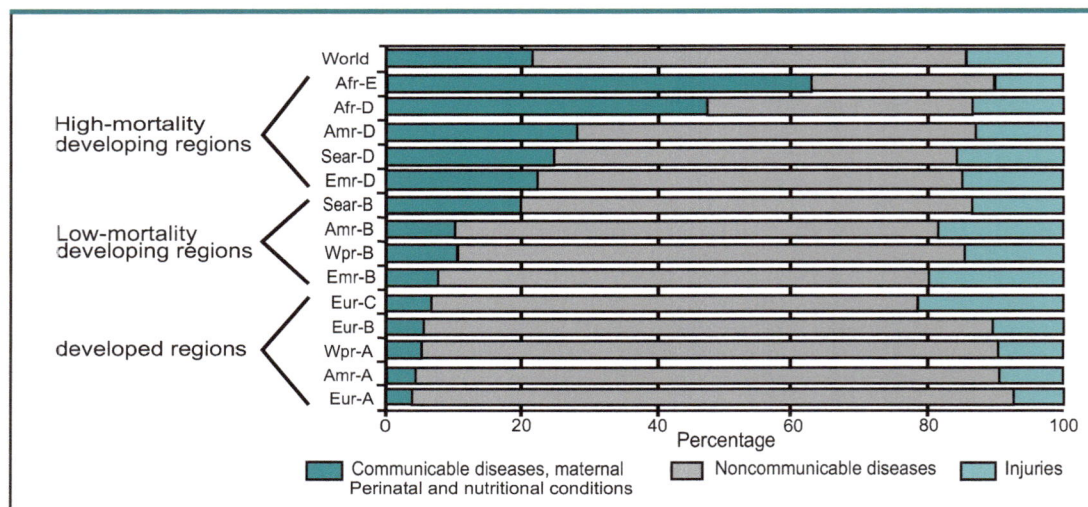

(Reproduced by kind permission of the World Health Organisation)

Figure 1. Deaths caused by different groups of diseases according to WHO regions.

3.2 Classification of Diabetes

3.2.1 A Simplified Definition

In simple terms, diabetes is a disorder in which the body becomes unable to control the amount of sugar in the blood. The pancreas (beta-cells) is not functioning normally, resulting in a partial or total lack of insulin or of its efficiency. Consequently, the system is no longer self-regulated and the level of sugar in the blood goes beyond the limits (threshold). The two main and common types of diabetes are Non Insulin Dependent Diabetes Mellitus (NIDDM) and Insulin Dependent Diabetes Mellitus (IDDM). The first type represents 75-90% of all diabetics, usually diagnosed after the age of 40 years and necessitating a treatment with diet alone or diet and tablets and ultimately insulin. The second type of diabetes is usually associated with younger people who need a treatment with insulin and diet.

3.2.2 Remark

Although with few medical precautions, Non Insulin Dependent Diabetes Mellitus is often called type 2 diabetes or adult diabetes. Similarly Insulin Dependent Diabetes Mellitus is called type 1 diabetes or juvenile diabetes or meagre diabetes. Other less frequent types of diabetes exist. For instance gestational diabetes is a kind of diabetes occurring in pregnant women.

Based on the Fasting glycaemia, diabetes is diagnosed according to the following concentrations of blood sugar:

Normal: Fasting glycaemia between 0.7-1.1 g/l

Pre-diabetes: Fasting glycaemia between 1.1-1.26 g/l

Diabetic: Fasting glycaemia greater than 1.26 g/l

3.3 Classification of Obesity and Overweight

The World Health Organisation (WHO) defines obesity as'' a condition of abnormal or excessive fat accumulation in adipose tissue, to the extent that health may be impaired''. The body fat being difficult to evaluate directly, a convenient measurement of obesity is given by the Body Mass Index (BMI) which is a simple weight to height ratio (kg/m^2). Accordingly, obesity in adults is defined as a BMI greater than $30 \ kg/m^2$ and international standards for classifying overweight and obesity worldwide are given (Table **2**). In children and adolescent, health professionals often use a BMI "growth chart" or BMI-for-age.

Table 2. Classification of overweight in adults according to BMI

Classification	BMI(kg/m^2)	Risk of co-morbidities
Underweight	<18.5	Low (but risk of other clinical problems increased)
Normal range	18.5 – 24.9	Average
Overweight	>25	
Pre-obese	25-29.9	Increased
Obese class I	30 – 34.9	Moderate
Obese class II	35 – 39.9	Severe
Obese class III	≥40	Very severe

3.4 Classification of Blood Pressure for Adults

A chronic high level of blood pressure, known as hypertension, constitutes a high risk for health. It is particularly associated with cardio vascular diseases. In order to reduce the burden of this condition, it is necessary to know the levels of normal and non normal blood pressure as given in Table **3**.

Table3. Classification of blood pressure for adults

Category	Systolic(mmHg)	Diastolic(mmHg)
Hypotension	<90	Or <60
Normal	90-119	And 60-79
Pre-hypertension	120-139	Or 80-89
Hypertension stage 1	140-159	Or 90-99
Hypertension stage 1	≥160	Or ≥100

4. MATERNAL MORTALITY

4.1 Maternal mortality

4.1.1 Concepts and definitions

Definition of maternal mortality: According to the International Statistical Classification of Diseases and Related Health Problems Tenth Revision, 1992(ICD-10), WHO defines maternal death as:

The death of a woman while pregnant or within 42 days of termination of pregnancy, irrespective of the duration and site of the pregnancy, from any cause related to or aggravated by the pregnancy or its management but not from accidental or incidental causes [4,5].

Alternative definition

Pregnancy-related death: The death of a woman while pregnant or within 42 days of termination of pregnancy, irrespective of the cause of death

Late maternal death: The death of a woman from direct or indirect obstetric causes, more than 42 days but less than one year after termination of pregnancy.

Measures of maternal mortality

Maternal mortality is often given by the crude numbers of deaths. The reading of these numbers, however, may be misleading when comparing two countries of different sizes. For instance: estimates for 2005 indicate that Japan had 70 maternal deaths and Guyana had 73. Based on these two crude numbers, the countries would have comparable maternal deaths, which is not true due to the population size in each country.

In order to overcome this inconvenience, standardized numbers are used.

Maternal Mortality Ratio: The most used indicator is the Maternal Mortality Ratio (MMR), defined as the number of maternal deaths in a population divided by the number of live births. This ratio also depicts the risk of maternal death relative to the number of births. If we go back to the precedent comparison, we find that MMR in Japan was 6 deaths per 100 000 live births compared to an MMR of 470 for Guyana.

Maternal Mortality Rate: Another indicator (apparently similar to, but actually different from MMR) is also used, it carries the name of Maternal Mortality Rate, defined as the number of maternal deaths in a population divided by the number of women of reproductive age. Besides reflecting the risk of maternal death per pregnancy or per birth (live birth or still-birth) this indicator takes into account the level of fertility in a population.

Lifetime risk of maternal mortality: Finally, adult lifetime risk of maternal mortality for women in the population can also be used as indicator. It is defined as the probability of dying from maternal cause during a woman's reproductive lifespan.

4.1.2 Remark

As expressed by the report released by the House of Commons International Development Committee in UK in 2008 [6], of all health measures, maternal mortality indicators represent the greatest gap between rich and poor countries. The gap between the two countries with the lowest and highest maternal mortality ratio was 1 over 2100 in 2005 (see chapter 4 on equity and diseases burden).

4.1.3 Example

Worldwide, maternal mortality rates vary considerably. Developed countries like Austria, Australia, Denmark, Germany, Greece, Iceland, Ireland, Italy, Spain, Sweden and Switzerland have an MMR less or equal to 5 deaths per 100 000 live births. At the opposite side, developing countries like Afghanistan, Angola, Burundi, Cameroon, Chad, Democratic Republic of Congo, Guinea-Bissau, Liberia, Malawi, Niger, Nigeria, Rwanda, Sierra Leone and Somalia have an MMR of at least 1000 deaths per 100 000 live births [7].

4.2 Infant mortality

4.2.1 Concepts and definitions

Neonatal mortality: Death of new born during the first 4 weeks of life.

Infant mortality: Death of children during the first year of life

Under five mortality: Death of children occurring before their fifth birthday.

As for maternal mortality, raw numbers may be used for neonatal, infant and under five deaths. However, in order to be able to compare mortality in countries with different sizes of population, crude numbers are "normalized" to give mortality rates.

Infant mortality rate is defined as the number of deaths of infants under one year of age per 1,000 live births in a given population. Neonatal and under five mortality rates are defined in a similar way.

4.2.2 Remarks

1. The accuracy of neonatal mortality may vary considerably depending on whether (or not) a country includes infants who die before the normal due date, also known as premature infants (miscarriages or natural abortions) and those who die during or immediately after childbirth, known as stillborn

2. Neonatal mortality accounts for 70% of infant mortality and more than half of all infants' deaths occur in the first week of life

4.2.3 Example

Worldwide, Neonatal Mortality Rates (NMR) vary considerably. Developed countries like Austria, Australia, Canada, Denmark, Finland, France, Germany, Greece, Iceland, Japan, Italy, Luxembourg, Monaco, Netherlands, New Zealand, Norway, Portugal, Spain, Sweden, Switzerland and United Kingdom have an NMR less or equal to 3 deaths per 1 000 live births. In contrast, developing countries like Afghanistan, Angola, Centre Africa, Cote d'Ivoire, Iraq, Lesotho, Liberia, Mali, Pakistan and Sierra Leone have an NMR of at least 50 deaths per 1000 live births [6,7]. A similar pattern is found when looking at Infant and Child Mortality rates [8]. It should be stressed, however, that few developing countries have low infant mortality comparable to the lowest levels achieved by developed countries. For instance Cuba (4) and Malaysia (5).

4.3 Morbidity

4.3.1 Concept of DALYs

In order to assess the impact of diseases and to facilitate meaningful comparisons of the disease burden across world regions, economic costs are often expressed in international dollars (an international dollar has the same purchasing power as one US dollar has in USA) and diseases are evaluated according to their burden in terms of mortality and disability. The most frequent method that has been used during the last decade is the approach that measures the disease burden in terms of disability adjusted life years (DALY) which is a combination of years of life lost (YLL) due to premature mortality, and years lived with disability (YLD). Thus, one DALY is thought of as one lost year of healthy life (either through death or illness/disability). Other metrics for disease burden can be found in the next chapters.

An average disability weight is affected to each disease according to the severity of its impact. As indicated in Table **4**, the weights vary between 0 (indicating full health) and 1(meaning death or equivalent) [9].

4.3.2 Example

Table 4. Average disability weight of selected diseases

Disease/cause/sequelae	Disability weight	Disease/cause/sequelae	Disability weight
Onchocerciasis -Blindness	0.600	Leprosy-Disabling	0.152
Onchocerciasis -Itching	0.068	Dengue Haemorrhagic Fever	0.210
Onchocerciasis –Low vision	0.260	Ascariasis- Contemporaneous Cognitive deficit	0.006
Trachoma -Blindness	0.600	Ascariasis-Cognitive impairment	0.463
Trachoma-Low vision	0.278	Ascariasis- Intestinal obstruction	0.024
Leishmaniasis-Visceral	0.243	Trichuriasis- Contemporaneous cognitive deficit	0.006
Leishmaniasis-Cutaneous	0.023	Trichuriasis- Massive dysentery syndrome	0.116
Schistosomiasis-Infection	0.006	Trichuriasis- Cognitive impairment	0.024

5. STRATEGIES AND EVALUATION

5.1 The Millennium Development Goals (MDGs)[10]

In September 2000, the international community adopted the Millennium Declaration expressing a strong commitment to universal development and poverty eradication (or at least reduction). Eight goals with specific targets were fixed and supposed to be reached by 2015 (Table **5**) [10].

Table 5. The Millennium Development Goals and targets

Goal	Target	Indicators
MDG1: Eradicate extreme poverty and hunger	Halve the % of people who suffer from hunger	Prevalence of underweight children under 5 years of age % population below minimum level of dietary energy consumption
MDG4: reduce child mortality	Reduce by 2/3 U5MR	Under5 mortality rate Infant mortality rate % of 1-year old children immunised against measles
MDG5: improve maternal health	Reduce by3/4 MMR	MMR % births attended by skilled health personnel
MDG6: Combat HIV/AIDS, malaria and other diseases	Have halted by 2015 and begun to reverse the spread of HIV/AIDS	HIV Prevalence among young people aged 15 to 24 Condom use contraceptive prevalence rate Number of children orphaned by HIV/AIDS
MDG7: Ensure environmental sustainability	Integrate the principles of sustainable development into country policies and programmes and reverse the loss of environment resources Halve by 2015 the % of people without sustainable access to safe drinking-water By 2020 to have achieved a significant improvement in the lives of at least 100 million slum dwellers	Proportion of population using solid fuel Proportion of population with sustainable access to improved water source, urban and rural Proportion of urban population with access to improved sanitation
MDG8: develop a global partnership for development	In cooperation with pharmaceutical companies, provide access to affordable essential drugs in developing countries	Proportion of population with access to affordable essential drugs on a sustainable basis
MDG2	Achieve universal primary education	Ensure that all boys and girls complete full course of primary education schooling
MDG3	Promote gender equality and empower women	Eliminate gender disparity in primary and secondary education preferably by 2005, and at all levels by 2015
MDG8	Develop a global partnership for development	

5.2 Cost-benefit and Cost-effective strategies

Cost-effective analysis (CEA) and cost-benefit analysis (CBA) are among the most used methods to evaluate programmes and health policies. The first method deals with the cost needed to reach a given health goal. For instance, how much it costs to reduce diabetes retinopathy by 30%, to reduce hypertension by 1mmHg, or a change in obesity by 20% BMI decrease in a given population. More generally, cost-effectiveness is measured by the cost per years of life saved or per DALYs yielded by a health action. The second method compares costs with benefits of a strategy. For example one US dollar invested in bed nets for malaria would yield a return of x US dollars gained from days of work saved.

A cost-benefit analysis by WHO showed that achievement of the MDG7 target in water and sanitation would allow for important economic gains. It was estimated that 1 US dollar invested would provide an economic return between 3 and 34 US dollars depending on regions. If the goal on water and sanitation were reached, reduction of diarrhoeal episodes by around 10% and the value of working days saved would yield More than 7 billion US dollars saved each year. In 2008, the Lancet published a series of three contributions devoted to chronic diseases in low-income and middle-income regions of the world. The third paper dealt with health effects and financial costs of strategies to reduce salt and control tobacco use. According to the authors of this paper, 23 countries have 80% of the burden of chronic disease in developing countries. In these countries, 13.8 million deaths could be averted over 10 years from 2006 to 2015(8.5 million by salt reduction strategy and 5.5 million by implementation of the WHO Framework Convention on Tobacco Control). The authors stated further that 75.6% of deaths averted would be from cardiovascular diseases, 15.4% would be from respiratory diseases and 8.7% from cancer. The strategies proposed were seen to be very cost-effective since the cost of their implementation would be less than US$0.40 per person per year in low-income and lower middle-income countries, and US$50-1.00 per person per year in upper middle-income countries (as of 2005) [11].

5.3 Child Development Index (CDI)

Stressing that millions of children are still denied proper healthcare, food, education and protection, Save the Children has consequently developed the Child Development Index (CDI) as a global multidimensional tool allowing to monitor how individual countries are performing in relation to the wellbeing of their children. The proposed index is based on three components: under-five mortality, underweight and non-enrolment in primary school (See next chapters for more details). Save the Children give regularly the CDI of different countries worldwide (Figure **2**).

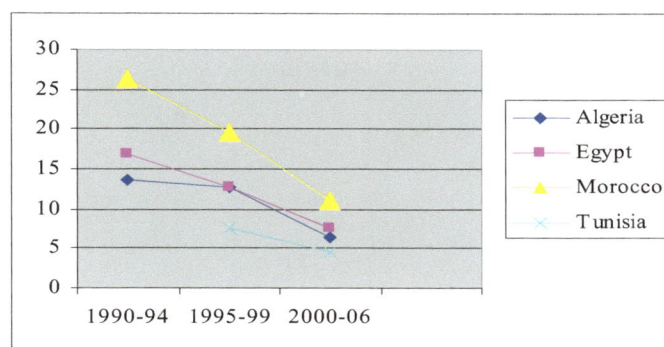

Figure 2. Evolution of Child Development Index in North Africa.

5.4 Basic Capability Index (BCI)

Considering that poverty is a multi-dimensional phenomenon needing a conceptual framework based on the rights of persons (and not on a markets), Social Watch has developed the Basic Capability Index as a way to identify poverty not based on income but rather based on internationally development goals in terms of education, children's health and reproductive health. The BCI is based on three indicators: percentage of children reaching fifth grade, survival until the fifth year of age and percentage of delivery assisted by skilled health personnel. Consequently, the highest possible BCI score is reached when all women receive medical assistance during labour, no child leaves school before completing the fifth grade and infant mortality is reduced to its lowest possible level of less than five deaths for every thousand.

5.4.1 Example

Morocco has a very low level (79), Egypt (88) is in the low level group, Algeria (94) and Tunisia (95) belong to the medium level class and Libya (98) is judged to have an acceptable level.

5.5 Concentration index

5.5.1 Definition

We plot the cumulative proportion of health outputs on the y-axis against the cumulative proportion of population at risk on the x-axis (starting with the most disadvantaged). If the curve coincides with the diagonal, it means that the outputs are the same for the whole population. The further the curve lays from the diagonal the greater the degree of inequality. The Concentration Index (noted C) is defined as twice the area between the concentration curve and the diagonal. The parameter C is between -1 and +1. The value C=-1 (respectively +1) indicates that health outputs are concentrated in the most disadvantaged people (respectively the least disadvantaged) (Figure **3**).

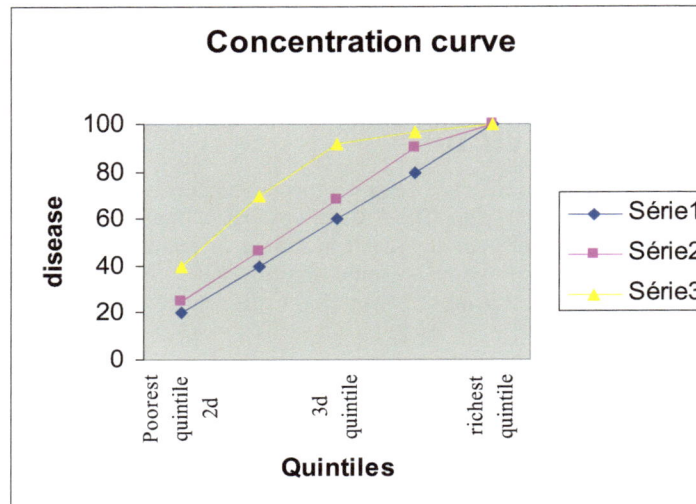

Figure 3. Concentration curves: an illustrative example.

The bleu line (diagonal) would be the ideal curve under perfect equity. The red curve represents a nearly equitable distribution. The yellow curve shows an inequitable distribution.

6. EQUITY: DEFINITIONS AND CONCEPTS

6.1 Definitions of equity / inequity

Equity in health has become a central issue. However, equity can mean different things to different people. Moreover, the principles underlying its definition and conceptualization may vary according to economic, medical, philosophical, political, ethical and other considerations. In what follows, we summarize few of the definitions found in literature on equity in health.

6.2 Health Equity as defined by the International Society of Equity in Health

Health equity is the absence of potentially remediable, systematic differences in one or more aspects of health across socially, economically, demographically, or geographically defined population groups or subgroups [12].

6.3 Health equity as defined in the Alma Ata Declaration

This Declaration strongly reaffirms that health, which is a state of complete physical, mental and social well being and not merely the absence of disease or infirmity, is a fundamental human right and that the attainment of the highest possible level of health is a most important world wide social goal whose realisation requires the action of many other social and economic sectors in addition to the health sector" [13].

6.4 Health equity as defined by the Commission on Social Determinants of Health

Where systematic differences in health are judged to be avoidable by reasonable action they are, quite simply, unfair. It is this that we label health inequity. Putting right theses inequalities -the huge and remediable differences in health between and within countries- is a matter of social justice. Reducing health inequities is an ethical imperative. Social injustice is killing people on grand scale [14].

6.5 Health equity as defined by Civil Society

Health is not a commodity but a public good. Health is an inalienable human right guaranteed by the United Nations and signed by all governments around the world more than six decades ago. The attainment of health does not revolve around bio-medical curative interventions alone, but basically on comprehensively addressing the structural social determinants of health including, but not limited to factors such as food security, safe water, sanitation, housing and working conditions. The major factors that hindered and continue to hinder the attainment of this goal and that increases the gap between people are the ruling neo-liberal paradigm of development led by and reflecting the narrow interests of the rich, of trans-national corporations and financial capital [15].

7. CONFLICT INTERSET

I declare that I have no conflict interest.

8. ACKNOWLEDGEMENTS

This paper was partly supported by a grant under the Global Project for Research (PGR) of the University Mohamed Premier, Oujda.

9. REFERENCES

1. The World Bank. [www.worldbank.gov Accessed 20/7/2009]
2. United Nations Development Programme [www.unds.org Accessed 20/7/2009]
3. WHO. The World Health Report 2003: Shaping the Future. World Health Organization Geneva, 2003a.
4. WHO. [www.who.int Accessed 20/7/2009]]
5. WHO: Maternal Mortality: estimated by WHO, UNICEF, UNFPA, and the World Bank. Geneva: World Heal(9th Organization 2007
6. House of Commons International Development Committee. Maternal Health: Fifth report of Session 2007-2008. London: The Stationery Office Limited 2007
7. WHO. The World Health Statistics 2008. World Health Organization Geneva, 2008.
8. Countdown Coverage Writing Group. Countdown to 2015 for maternal, newborn, and child survival: the 2008 report on tracking coverage of interventions. Lancet 2008; 371: 1247-1258
9. Boutayeb A. Developing countries and neglected diseases: challenges and perspectives. Int. J. Eq. Health 2007 doi: 10.1186/1475-927 – 6-20
10. UN. United Nations Millennium Declaration. New York, NY, United Nations, 2000
11. Asaria P, Chisholm D, Mathers C, Ezzati M, Beaglehole R. Chronic disease prevention: health effects and financial costs of strategies to reduce salt intake and control tobacco use. Lancet 2008; 370:2044-53.
12. ISEqH [www.equityhealthj.com/definitions Accessed 21/7/2009]
13. Declaration of Alma-Ata. International Conference on primary health care, Alma-Ata, USSR, 6.12 September 1978. Geneva, World Health Organization, 1978
14. Commission on Social Determinants of health. Closing the gap in a generation: health equity through action on the social determinants of health. Geneva: World Health Organization, 2008
15. Civil Society 2008, Social Medicine 2008, **2** (4), 192-211].

CHAPTER 2

Health Risks: Illustrating the Link between Social Determinants, Health Equity and Development

Abdesslam Boutayeb

Department of Mathematics Faculty of Sciences, Boulevard Mohamed VI, BP: 717 Oujda, Morocco;
Email: x.boutayeb@menara.ma

Abstract: Between and within countries, disadvantaged people are the most affected by health risks globally. Underweight, micronutrients deficiency, lack of hygiene, unsafe water, inadequate sanitation, work and road accidents, violence and sex abuse, are clearly more prevalent among children, women, elderly, poor and less educated people, workers with low occupations, and other discriminated groups on the basis of ethnicity, culture, religion, and other. More globally, under nutrition, overweight, blood pressure, high cholesterol, tobacco, alcohol, illicit drugs, low fruits and vegetables intake, physical inactivity, unsafe sex, work injuries, road accidents, violence and environmental hazards constitute important health risks which illustrate the link between social determinants, health equity and development. Millions of deaths and tens of millions of disability years can be saved by tackling these factors worldwide in general and in developing countries in particular.

Keywords: Risk Factor, Tobacco, diet, alcohol, physical activity, injury, accident, blood pressure, unsafe sex.

1. INTRODUCTION

Health risks are the most illustrative factors of the link between social determinants, health equity and development. The most common risks are: under nutrition, overweight, blood pressure, high cholesterol, tobacco, alcohol, illicit drugs, low fruits and vegetables intake, physical inactivity, unsafe sex, work injuries, road accidents, violence and environmental hazards [1,2].

The relation is often so complicated that it is difficult to distinguish the cause from the consequence. For example, on the one hand, under-nutrition can be seen as a direct consequence of lack of economic development and/or inequity in health. On the other hand, under-nutrition makes people more exposed to death and infections, reduces life expectancy and quality of life, and hence affects human capital and causes under development.

Between and within countries, disadvantaged people are the most affected by health risks globally. Underweight, micronutrients deficiency, lack of hygiene, unsafe water, inadequate sanitation, work and road accidents, violence and sex abuse, are clearly affecting children, women, elderly, poor and less educated people, workers with low occupations, and other discriminated groups on the basis of ethnicity, culture, religion, and other. Moreover, these health risks interact, accumulate and lead to the vicious cycle of inequality traps (see chapter). In addition, although to a less extent, disadvantaged people also share the burden of other risk factors more commonly associated with the well off (blood pressure, overweight, fruit and vegetable intake, physical inactivity, tobacco, alcohol, illicit drugs and others). For example, obesity and tobacco consumption are initially found among the non-impoverished within regions, and later these risks are given up by the non-impoverished but taken up among the impoverished [3].

On top of the millions of deaths they cause annually, health risks also engender millions of Disability Adjusted Life Years (DALYs) (Table 1).

Table 1. Burden disease and risk factors worldwide in 1990 and 2001(in millions)

Risk factor	DALYs (1990)	% of total DALYS	DALYs (2001)	% of total DALYs
Underweight	220	15.9	138	9.5
Poor water, hygiene, sanitation	93	6.8	54	3.7
Unsafe sex	49	3.5	92	6.3
Alcohol	48	3.5	58	4.0
Occupation	38	2.7	23	1.6
Tobacco	36	2.6	59	4.1

Risk factor	DALYs (1990)	% of total DALYS	DALYs (2001)	% of total DALYs
Blood Pressure	19	1.4	64	4.5
Physical inactivity	14	1.0	27	1.9
Illicit drugs	8	0.6	11	0.7
Air pollution	7	0.5	19	1.3

2. HEALTH RISKS

2.1 Under nutrition

Defined in public health by poor anthropometric status (weight, height,..), under nutrition and malnutrion are often used interchangeably to indicate inadequate diet characterized by deficiencies in calories, protein and/or various micronutrients. In low-income countries, poverty constitutes an obvious underlying determinant of global deficiency in nutrition. The last figures released by FAO on poverty are alarming [4,5]. In 2009, worldwide, more than one billion people are undernourished, amounting to one sixth of all humanity and representing an increase of 100 million as compared to 2008. Although the current economic crisis makes the rising hunger as a global phenomenon sweeping the whole world, the burden of hunger is affecting differently the world regions and various groups in each region. More than 90% of the population suffering from hunger live in Sub-Saharan Africa (32% of its population), and Asia and Pacific. The near East and North Africa region has known the largest percentage increase in developing countries (+13.5%). The phenomenon is, however, not restricted to developing countries, since hunger has increased by 15.4% in developed countries (Figure **1**).

The repercussion of poverty on health is straightforward. First of all, households cannot afford meat, dairy products, fruits and vegetables, and other protein- and nutrient-rich foods and hence their expenditure is more directed to cheaper food like grains. Secondly, poor women are less likely to seek health care for themselves or their children. Thirdly, poverty increases the number of street children who withdraw prematurely from school, including homeless and working children. Finally, more globally, lack of income yields violence, suicide and other mental diseases. It should be stressed that, however, between and within regions, disadvantaged people are always the groups who suffer more from poverty and consequently from ill-health.

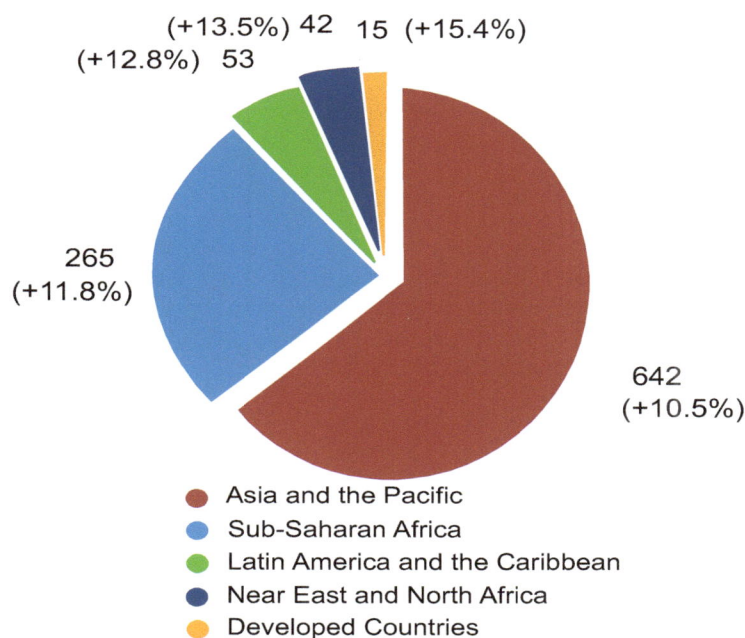

Figure 1. Estimated regional distribution of hunger (in million) and increase from 2008 levels (in %). Printed with kind permission of the Food and Agriculture Organization (FAO) of the United Nations.

In middle-income countries and affluent countries, inadequate diet is rather expressed as malnutrition, in the sense that, despite sufficient households' income, some people may suffer from deficiency of vitamin, iron, iodine, calcium, zinc and other necessary nutrients. The World Health Report 2002 devoted the chapter 4 to the quantification of selected major risks to health [3]. The report indicated that around the year 2000, vitamin and nutrients deficiency affected large proportions of population worldwide. For instance, it was estimated that nearly one third of the world population was at risk or suffered from iron, zinc and iodine deficiency, and one fifth of the population was in need of vitamin A. The burden of these deficiencies was expressed in millions of deaths and tens of millions of DALYS (Table **2**).

Table 2. Vitamin and micronutrients deficiency

Risk factor	Vitamin A deficiency	Iron deficiency	Iodine deficiency	Zinc deficiency
Prevalence	21%	2 billion people	2.2 billion at risk 1 billion goitre	1/3 of the world population
Region most affected	South East Asia & Africa	Africa, South East Asia, West Pacific	Africa, South East Asia Eastern Mediterranean region	Africa, South East Asia Eastern Mediterranean region
Population at highest risk	Children, women of reproductive age	Young children, pregnant and post-partum women	adults	All categories
Associated health	Mental, vision, growth, immunity	Anaemia, mental retardation	Brain damage, mental retardation	Lower respiratory track, malaria, diarrhoeal disease
Deaths caused	0.8 million (1.4%)	0.8 million (1.5%)		0.8 million (1.4%)
DALYs caused	22.5 million (1.8%)	35 million (2.4%)	2.5 million (0.2%)	28 million (2.9%)

Globally, in 2000, underweight caused 3.7 million deaths of which about 1.8 million deaths in Africa. Moreover, beyond mortality figures, underweight is also responsible for important morbidity, causing nearly 10% of the total DALYs.

Although all ages are at risk of being underweight, children and women of reproductive age are particularly at high risk. In 2000, the World Health Organization estimated that approximately 27% (168 million) of children under five years of age were underweight around the world. The distribution is, however, uneven and reveals high levels of inequity. Indeed, child underweight increases significantly with the level of poverty. The risk of underweight in people living on less than $1 per day is two- to three-fold higher than for those living on more than $2 per day.

2.2 Low Fruit and Vegetables Intake

According to the WHO report 2002 [1], nearly 5% of deaths (2.7 million) and nearly 2% (27 million) DALYs were attributable to low fruit and vegetable intake. This health risk caused nearly 20% of gastrointestinal cancer, about 31% of ischaemic heart disease, and 11% of stroke worldwide. More globally, about 85% of this burden was caused by cardiovascular diseases and 15% by cancer [5].

Healthy diet in general and consumption of fruit and vegetable in particular, varies according to the level of income as indicated by a recent report devoted to a critical analysis of public health policies in eight European countries [6]. This report indicates that in England, nearly 40% of women from the highest income quintile were eating 5 or more portions of fruit and vegetables per day compared to less than 20% of women in the lowest income quintile. In Sweden, only 5% of men and 14 of women aged 18-84 years reported that they ate the equivalent of 500 grams of fruit/vegetables per day in 2006.

2.3 Physical Inactivity

Worldwide, physical inactivity was globally estimated to cause nearly 2 million deaths and 20 million DALYs in 2001. In particular, from 10 to 16% of cases of breast cancer, colon and rectal cancers, and diabetes, and about 20% of ischaemic heart disease were attributable to this risk factor.

Although, there is no internationally agreed definition allowing to quantify the needed physical activity, all reports indicate that the present levels of activity should be enhanced.

In Sweden, around 1/3 of all adults exercise less than the recommended amount of 30muniutes per day and 14% of the population reported being sedentary in their spare time. However, sedentary lifestyle was more common for those who have not attained an upper secondary education and eating habits were seen to vary between different cultural and social backgrounds [6].

2.4 "Overnutrition"

Beside the problems caused by under nutrition, under physical activity and low fruit and vegetables intake, and lack of access to safe water, and adequate sanitation, a substantial part of the disease burden can be attributed to high pressure, high levels of sugar and cholesterol, mainly due to over consumption of fatty food, carbohydrates, salt, alcohol, tobacco, additives substances, etc…

2.5 Overweight/Obesity

The World Health Organisation (WHO) defines obesity as "a condition of abnormal or excessive fat accumulation in adipose tissue, to the extent that health may be impaired" [5]. The body fat being difficult to evaluate directly, a convenient measurement of obesity is given by the Body Mass Index (BMI) which is a simple weight to height ratio (kg/m^2). Accordingly, obesity in adults is defined as a BMI greater than 30 kg/m^2 and international standards for classifying overweight and obesity worldwide are given (See chapters 1&5). In children and adolescent, health professionals often use a BMI "growth chart" or BMI-for-age (see WHO Reference 2007: http://www.who.int/growthref/en/).

However, it should be stressed that BMI may miss some aspects of obesity like the regional distribution of excess body fat in general and excessive abdominal fat in particular. The last form, known as central obesity, is more indicated as a risk for type 2 diabetes.

Worldwide, overweight and obesity affect 1.2 billion of which 300 million are clinically obese. In some developed countries like the USA, the prevalence reaches 60%. But developing countries like those of the Middle East have also a very high prevalence. There is especially two features that needs serious reflection: the first one is a concern about the growing prevalence of obesity in children since it is estimated that 10% of the world's children are overweight or obese; the second is the fact that many developing countries are now facing the coexistence of under- and overweight people [7,8,9].

The last two decades have seen a dramatic increase in overweight and obesity rates all over the world, although with some differences between and within countries. This alarming trend is linked to a number of factors, including genetic, gender and socio-economic status. Many transition forms (epidemiological, democratic, demographic, ..) have been suspected but the most established link is with the transition from a rural to an urban lifestyle and its corollary of nutrition transition characterised by a higher energy density diet with a greater role for fat and added sugar in foods, greater saturated fat intake mostly from animal sources (Table **4**), reduced intakes of complex carbohydrates and fibres, and reduced fruit and vegetables; with a decrease in physical activity.

Classified as a disease, obesity diminishes both quality of life and life expectancy, but it is also a common risk factor for other diseases like CVDs, arthritis, type 2 diabetes and many types of cancer. According to the International Obesity Task Force (IOTF) and the WHO World Health report 2002 [3], about 60% of diabetes, 20% of ischaemic heart disease, and 8-40% of certain cancers can be attributable to overweight and obesity. More generally, obesity diminishes the quality of life and increases risks of morbidity (Table **3**).

Table 3. Classification of overweight in adults according to BMI

Classification	BMI(kg/m^2)	Risk of co-morbidities
Underweight	<18.5	Low(but risk of other clinical problems increased)
Normal range	18.5 – 24.9	Average
Overweight	>25	
Pre-obese	25-29.9	Increased
Obese class I	30 – 34.9	Moderate
Obese class II	35 – 39.9	Severe
Obese class III	≥40	Very severe

2.6 Tobacco

Among all avoidable risks to health, tobacco is the number one enemy, causing every year more than 5 million deaths and some 60 million DALYS(4.5% of total DALYs) [2,5,10](Table **4**). The deaths from tobacco-associated diseases such as cancer, chronic lung disease, diabetes and CVDs, cumulated approximately 100 million deaths during the twentieth century. More than 50% of the 5 million deaths attributed to smoking in 2000 occurred in developing countries, where smoking prevalence among men is nearly 50%. Curiously, while tobacco consumption is falling in the most developed countries, it is increasing in developing countries by about 3.4% per annum. Despite the repeated calls regularly launched by researchers and humanitarian organizations stressing the dramatic consequences of tobacco, the majority of developing countries which signed the Framework Convention on Tobacco Control (FCTC) are not applying any measure to control smoking at least in public areas [11].

Table 4. Burden disease and risk factors worldwide year2002 (in millions)

Risk factor	Deaths (1990)(x10^3)	% of total deaths	DALYs (2001))(x10^3)	% of total DALYs
Hypertension	7141	12.8	64270	04.5
Tobacco	4907	08.8	59081	04.1
Unsafe sex	4415	07.9	40437	02.8
High cholesterol	2726	04.9	26662	01.9
Low fruit & vegetables	2591	04.6	33415	02.3
Alcohol	1804	03.2	58323	04.0
Physical inactivity	1922	03.4	19092	01.3

2.7 Alcohol

Worldwide, about 2 million deaths were attributable to alcohol in 2000. Its consumption has known an increasing trend during the last decades, especially in low-income and middle-income countries. Alcohol is estimated to cause 20 to 30% of esophagus cancer, liver disease, epilepsy, motor vehicle accidents and other hazards, amounting globally to 4% of the global disease burden.

2.8 Road Accidents

Worldwide, every year, road accidents cause more than 1.2 million deaths and between 20 and 50 million non-fatal injuries. The burden of road accidents is mainly born by low-income and middle-income countries, where 90% of the world's fatalities occur. Although low-income and middle income countries have only 48% of the world's vehicles, the rates of road traffic fatality in these two country groups are 21.5 and 19.5 respectively per 100 000 population compared to 10.3 per 100 000 population in high-income countries.

Pedestrians, cyclists and those riding motorised two-or three-wheelers constitute the most vulnerable groups.

According to WHO's Global Burden of Disease Project for 2004, road traffic caused over 1.27 million deaths that year.

In 2004, road traffic injuries were at the ninth rank of leading causes of deaths, responsible of 2.2 of the whole burden. If the present trend is maintained, it is expected that road traffic injuries will jump to the fifth rank in 2030, causing 3.6% of the total deaths.

2.9 Child Injury

Every year, injuries and violence kill nearly one million children (aged less than 18 years). 95% of deaths caused by child injuries occur in low-income and middle-income countries.

According to a UNICEF report, child injuries declined by 50% in high-income countries between 1970 and 1995 in contrast to an increasing trend in low-income countries.

The Global Childhood Unintentional Injury Surveillance (GCUIS) study launched in 2007 in four countries (Bangladesh, Colombia, Egypt,and Pakistan) based on children less than 11 years of age showed that 63% of injuries occurred in leisure/play time, 11% during travels, 9% in daily living, 5% at work (paid or unpaid), 4% in sports and 3%, in educational activity. Road traffic injuries accounted for 22% of all injuries (39% pedestrians, 19% passengers, 13% motorcycle or moped riders [12].

According to a study comparing outcomes of severely injured patients in three countries of different economic levels showed that case-fatality rates among seriously injured persons (injury severity score greater than 9) was 35% in the high-income country (USA), 55% in middle-income country (Mexico) and 63% in low-income country Ghana. These figures clearly indicate that, for a similar level of severe injury, patients in low-income countries are twice likely to die than those from high-income countries. The authors state that elimination of these inequities could avert 2 million of the 5 million injury deaths every year [13].

3. CONFLICT INTERSET

I declare that I have no conflict interest

4. ACKNOWLEDGEMENTS

This paper was partly supported by a grant under the Global Project for Research (PGR) of the University Mohamed Premier, Oujda.

5. REFERENCES

1.   WHO. The World health report: Reducing Risk: Promoting Health Life. Geneva, World Health Organization. [http://www.who.int/whr/2002/en].
2.   Boutayeb A. The double burden of communicable and non communicable diseases in developing countries. Transactions of the Royal Society of Tropical Medicine and Hygiene 2006; 100:191-199
3.   WHO. The World Health Report 2002 http://www.who.int/whr/2002/en/whr02_ch4.pdf].
4.   FAO. More people than ever are victims of hunger[www.fao.org accessed 1/1/2009]
5.   World Health Organisation: Diet, Nutrition and the prevention of Chronic Diseases. In Technical report Series 916 Geneva, World Health Organization; 2003.
6.   Hogsted C, Moberg H, uLundgren B, Backhans M. Health for all? A critical analysis of public health polices in eight European countries. Swedish National Institute of Public Health, 2009.
7.   Boutayeb A, Boutayeb S. The brden of non communicable diseases in developing countries. Int. J. Equity Health 2005, doi:10.1186/1475-9276-4-2
8.   Drewnowski, A., Specter, S.E., 2004. Poverty and obesity: The role of energy density and energy costs. Am. J. Clin. Nutr. 79, 6—16.
9.   Kenchaiah S, Evans JC, Levy D, Wilson PM, Benjamin EJ, Larson MG et al. Obesity and the risk of heart failure. N Engl J Med 2002, 347:305-313.
10. WHO, 2000. This month's special theme: Tobacco. Bull. World Health Organ. 78, part 7.
11. Joossens L: From public health to international law: possible protocols for inclusion in the Framework Convention on Tobacco Control. Bulletin of the World Health Organization 2000, 78:930-937.
12. Hyder AA, Sugerman DE, Puvanachandra P et al. Global childhood unintentional injury surveillance in four cities in developing countries: a pilot study. Bull World Health Organ 2009;87:345-352
13. Mock C, Abantanga F, Goosen J, Joshipura M, Juillard C. Strengthening care of injured children globally. Bull World Health Organ 2009;87:382-389

CHAPTER 3

A Decade of Equity: A Selection of Recent Bibliography on Equity and Social Determinants of Health

Abdesslam Boutayeb[1,*] and Saber Boutayeb[2]

[1]*Department of Mathematics Faculty of Sciences, Boulevard Mohamed VI, BP: 717 Oujda, Morocco;*
Email: x.boutayeb@menara.ma

[2]*Institut National d'Oncologie Service Oncologie Médicale, Rabat, Morocco;*
Email: boutayebdr@yahoo.fr

Abstract: Equity in health has become a central issue. However, equity can mean different things to different people. Moreover, the principles underlying its definition and conceptualization may vary according to economic, medical, philosophical, political, ethical and other considerations. During the last decades, the literature on health equity has known an exponential increase. Although the majority of publications are produced in developed countries, the part devoted to developing countries is rapidly increasing

This chapter is dedicated to a selection of recent papers published on equity and social determinants underlying it. Our intention is not to give an exhaustive panorama of all papers which dealt with the theme of equity, rather we have selected some of the papers that could help the reader to easily get an overview of the multidimensional aspects of equity as illustrated by the large number of publications dealing with definitions and concepts of equity, the difference between inequalities and inequities, inequity in access to health services and health status, and many other aspects.

For each paper cited, we have tried to summarise the method used, the main results and the conclusion. When a detailed abstract was available, we have used it in a slightly different and concise form.

The papers reviewed were grouped into sub topics:

1. Definitions and Concepts, 2. Social determinants of Health, 3. Diseases and equity, 4. Equity and children health, 5. Maternal health and violence, 6. Geographic disparity, 7. Migrants and heath equity, 8. Equity and finance.

Keywords: Health (in)equity, developed countries, developing countries, measurements, social determinants, diseases, maternal, infant, tool, concept.

1. INTRODUCTION

Equity in health has become a central issue. However, equity can mean different things to different people. Moreover, the principles underlying its definition and conceptualization may vary according to economic, medical, philosophical, political, ethical and other considerations. During the last decades, the literature on health equity has known an exponential increase. Although the majority of publications are produced in developed countries, the part devoted to developing countries is rapidly increasing.

In the world health report 2000, devoted entirely to health systems and the way of improving their performance, the World Health Organization expanded its traditional concern for people's physical and mental well-being to emphasize other elements such as goodness and fairness.

The report stated that "while improving health is clearly the main objective of a health system, it is not the only one. The objective of good health itself is really twofold: the best attainable average level goodness – and the smallest feasible differences among individuals and groups – Fairness". According to this report, goodness means a health system responding well to what people expect of it and fairness means it responds equally well to everyone, without discrimination [1].

---

*Corresponding author

Since its publication, however, the report's approach to measuring inequalities has been criticized by several authors. Most of them argued that the WHO approach measures inequalities across individuals instead of considering inequity between social groups.

In the constitution adopted in June 2000, at the Inaugural Conference of the International Society for Equity in Health (ISEqH), equity in health was defined as "The absence of systematic and potentially remediable differences in one or more aspects of health across populations or population groups defined socially, economically, demographically, or geographically"[2]. It was further stressed that the purpose for which ISEqH is formed is to promote equity in health and in health care services internationally through education, research, publication and communication. These objectives are being achieved to a certain extent by the International Journal for Equity in Health, the official journal of ISEqH.

Launched in March 2005, the WHO Commission on the Social Determinants of Health (WHO-CSDH) has delivered its important report in 2008 "Closing the gap in a generation" [3]. According to this report, the poorest of the poor have high levels of illness and premature mortality. But poor health is not confined to those worst off. In countries at all levels of income, health and illness follow a social gradient: the lower the socioeconomic position, the worse the health. Between countries, a dramatic illustration is given by the gap in life expectancy at birth, varying from more than 80 years in some developed countries to less than 50 years in several African countries. The Commission stresses that "Where systematic differences in health are judged to be avoidable by reasonable action, they are, quite simply, unfair. It is this that we label health inequity".

In parallel, the report released by Civil Society in 2008 underlined that Health is not a commodity but a public good which constitutes an inalienable human right guaranteed by the United Nations and signed by all governments around the world more than six decades ago. It was further emphasized that the attainment of health does not revolve around bio-medical curative interventions alone, but basically on comprehensively addressing the structural social determinants of health including, but not limited to factors such as food security, safe water, sanitation, housing and working conditions. This report stresses, amongst other, that an estimated 30 000 children die every day, mainly from preventable and easily treatable disease; what is important is not just that so many children die unnecessarily, but also that they die in much larger numbers in certain regions of the world, and within regions, in certain communities [4].

Complementing the work of the WHO-CSDH and building on the work of a previous project "Closing the Gap (2004-2007)", the European Union has created "DETERMINE (2007-2010)" as a wide initiative to stimulate action on the social and economic determinants of health inequity, bringing together a Consortium of over 50 health bodies, public health and health promotion institutes, governments and various other organizations from 26 European countries [5].

The World Bank, in its World Development Report 2006 defines equity in terms of opportunities: "By equity we mean that individuals should have equal opportunities to pursue a life of their choosing and be spared from extreme deprivation in outcomes" [6]. The World Bank's Reaching the Poor Program(RPP) was initiated as a response to the findings of a previous Bank's research, affirming that health services intended for the poor were in fact not reaching the poor but rather benefiting to the well off. It should be stressed, however, that World Bank endorses a large responsibility in exacerbating inequity in developing countries through the well known structural adjustment programmes of the 1980s. According to this report, the second set of reasons why equity and long-term prosperity can be complementary arises from the fact that high levels of economic and political inequality tend to lead to economic institutions and social arrangements that systematically favour the interests of those with more influence. The adverse effects of unequal opportunities and political power on development are all the more damaging because economic, political, and social inequalities tend to reproduce themselves over time and across generations. The authors of this report call such phenomenal "inequality traps".

Worldwide, only 10% of all resources for health research is spent on diseases that account for 90% of the total global disease burden. The Global Forum for Health Research (GFHR) was created in 1998 with the main goal "helping correct the 10/90 gap". The Forum celebrated 10 years of working for research for the health of the poor by devoting several conferences and publications to equity in health access and health status [7].

Among the various activities of the International Union for Scientific Studies in Populations (IUSSP), a Scientific Panel on "Health Equity and Policy in the Arab World" was launched in 2006 in order to organize different seminars preparing for the International Population Conference to be held in September 2009 [8].

This large "movement towards equity" has particularly interested the scientific community which increased the number of publications on equity during the last decades, trying to give more precise and sophisticated definitions, and to understand the causes of the causes and pathways through which in(equity) arises.

This chapter is dedicated to a selection of recent papers published on equity and social determinants underlying it. Our intention is not to give an exhaustive panorama of all papers which dealt with the theme of equity, rather we have selected some of the papers that could help the reader to easily get an overview of the multidimensional aspects of equity as illustrated by the large number of publications dealing with definitions and concepts of equity, the difference between inequalities and inequities, inequity in access to health services and health status, and many other aspects.

For each paper cited, we have tried to summarise the method used, the main results and the conclusion. When a detailed abstract was available, we have used it in a slightly different and concise form.

The papers reviewed were grouped into sub topics:

1. Definitions and Concepts, 2. Social determinants of Health, 3. Diseases and equity, 4. Equity and children health, 5. Maternal health and violence, 6. Geographic disparity, 7. migration and equity, 8. Equity and finance

2. DEFINITIONS AND CONCEPTS

Many authors have tried to stress the difference between (in)equity and (in)equality. In fact, inequalities are not all inequities. For example, men and women are biologically different but the difference is not an inequity. In counterpart, when in the same society, women receive less education, are underpaid and/or have limited access to political and socioeconomic responsibilities, the matter becomes unjust and hence inequality between men and women is well established as an inequity.

Health differences and inequalities are usually described by dividing the population into sub groups where the differences are engendered by variables such as sex, age, social status, ethnicity and geographic area. More precision on the differences may be provided by breaking down each variable. For instance, socio economic status may give various stratifications according to levels of income, education, professional occupation, material assets, etc...

In 2000 a special issue of the Bulletin of the World Health Organization was devoted to the theme of inequalities in health, covering topics like poverty and inequity: a proper focus for the new century [9], public spending on health in Africa: do the poor benefit? [10], health inequalities and the health of the poor: what we know? What can we do [11], socioeconomic inequalities in child mortality: comparisons across nine developing countries [12], defining and measuring health inequality: an approach based on the distribution of health expectancy [13]. The discussion and debate on defining and measuring health equity continued through other issues of the bulletin [14-16]. In particular, the WHO report 2000 and its approach to measuring inequality was criticised by several authors. Most of them argued that the WHO approach measures inequalities across individuals instead of considering inequity between social groups. The two following papers were published in this sprit [17, 18].

Braveman P, Starfield B, Geiger H Jack. World Health Report 2000: how it removes equity from the agenda for public health monitoring and policy. BMJ 2001; 323(7314): 678–681

In this paper, while applauding the recommendation made in the WHO Report 2000 to assess national health systems not only by the average health status of a country's population but also by the extent to which health varies within the population, the authors argue that the report's measure of health inequalities is not useful for guiding national policy because it provides no information to guide resource allocation or to target policies. In addition, it does not measure socioeconomic or other social disparities in health within countries. The authors add that, when used as a substitute for monitoring social inequalities in health, it removes equity and human rights considerations from the routine measurement and reporting of health disparities within nations. As a support to their arguments, the authors compared the rankings based on the World Health Report 2000 measure of inequalities in child survival for 44 countries with available data, with rankings using the poor/rich ratio and the concentration index [17].

Asada Y, Hedemann T. A Problem with the Individual Approach in the WHO Health Inequality Measurement. Int J Equity Health 2002 [http://www.equityhealthj.com/content/1/1/2]

Criticizing the controversial choice used in the World Health Report 2000 to measure inequality across individuals rather than across groups, the authors have dealt with three questions: (1) is the World Health Organization's health inequality measure value-free as it claims? (2) if it is not, what is the normative position implied by its approach when measuring health inequality? and (3) is the individual approach a logically consistent methodological choice for that normative position? In conclusion, the authors agued that the World Health Organization's health inequality measure is not value-free. If it was, the health inequality information that the measurement collected could not reasonably be included in its ranking of how well national health systems performed. The World Health Organization's normative position can be interpreted as a quite expansive view of justice, in which health distributions that have causes amenable to human intervention are considered to be matters of justice [18].

During the 1980s, the World Bank imposed its well known structural adjustment programmes to most developing countries where social sectors were considered as non productive and hence marginalised. Consequently, the World Bank assumes a large part of responsibility in actual inequities in low- and middle-income countries. By the dawn of the third millennium, however, the World Bank seemed to have shifted its policy towards more equity in poor countries. The World Report 2006 and the book based on individual country reports show the interest of the World Bank in equity.

The World Bank. World Development Report 2006[www.worlbank.org]

In this report it is said that "By equity we mean that individuals should have equal opportunities to pursue a life of their choosing and be spared from extreme deprivation in outcomes. The main message is that equity is complementary, in some fundamental respects, to the pursuit of long-term prosperity". The report relates the experience of two countries: Spain which has gone from authoritarianism and under-development to democracy and wealth by combining equity and development in the transition to democracy, and Indonesia which achieved at the same time growth, equity and poverty reduction. It also discusses among others, the phenomenon of "inequality traps" explained as follows: Disadvantaged children from families at the bottom of the wealth distribution do not have the same opportunities as children from wealthier families to receive quality education. So these disadvantaged children can expect to earn less as adults. Because the poor have less voice in the political process, they -like their parents- will be less able to influence spending decisions to improve public schools for their children. And the cycle of underachievement continues [6].

Gwatkin DR, Rutstein S, Johnson K, Suliman E, Wagstaff A, Amouzou A. Socio-Economic Differences in Health, Nutrition, and Population within Developing Countries: An Overview. The World Bank 2007 HNP

This book by Gwatkin *et al* gathers invaluable information on health inequities. It gives an overview based on 56 individual reports produced in low-income and middle-income countries where data was available through Demographic and Health Surveys (DHS). The book analyses health and nutrition determinants and health status, disaggregating data by quintiles of wealth or household assets [19]. Multidimensional aspects of inequity are considered through morbidity and mortality, immunisation coverage, nutritional status, micronutrients, access to health services, education, domestic violence, antenatal and postnatal care, delivery assistance, contraception, and others. Despite the critics addressed to this document in using for instance a single indicator such as asset indices and asset quintiles which do not fully address inequities conferred by age, gender, ethnic group, or position within the household family structure, this book remains an important source for comparisons within and between countries in terms of inequalities and inequities. Moreover, the book can be complemented by the 56 individual country reports available at http://www.worldbank.org/povertyandhealth/countrydata

The International Society for Equity in Health was formed with the purpose to promote equity in health and in health care services internationally through education, research, publication and communication. These objectives are being achieved to a certain extent by the International Journal for Equity in Health, the official journal of ISEqH. Indeed, this online and free accessible journal constitutes a forum for research on equity and related topics, providing health researchers with interesting and diverse publications. However, this journal in not alone in this scientific and humanitarian run towards the promotion of equity, and a multitude of other journals publish papers on equity (although with a less frequency).

To start with, the reader is refereed to the first paper published in IJEqH on annotated bibliography on equity in health from 1980 to 2001.

Macinko JA, Starfield B. Annotated Bibliography on Equity in Health, 1980-2001 Measuring total health inequality: adding individual variation to group-level differences. Int J Equity Health 2002 [http://www.equityhealthj.com/content/1/1/1]

The purposes of this bibliography are to present an overview of the published literature on equity in health and to summarize key articles relevant to the mission of the International Society for Equity in Health (ISEqH). The intent is to show the directions being taken in health equity research including theories, methods, and interventions to understand the genesis of inequities and their remediation. Therefore, the bibliography includes articles from the health equity literature that focus on mechanisms by which inequities in health arise and approaches to reducing them where and when they exist [20].

Many authors have dealt with the crucial problem of measuring health inequalities either through theoretical lenses or directly on the field at local, national and international levels.

The following contributions are cited by order 1) theory and tools, 2) Globalisation and equity 3) regional level, 4) national level.

2.1 Theory and tools

The importance of equity in health necessitates concise definitions of concepts and tools used either to describe the distribution of ill-health as a phenomenon in time and space, or to understand the causes underlying unfair and avoidable inequalities in order to act on them. Consequently, the measures of health inequalities depend on the approach adopted to distinguish different groups of a population (by sex, socioeconomic status, education level, residence area, income, ethnic groups,...), the health variable to be described (mortality, morbidity, expectancy, quality of life, nutrition, access to services, ...), and the methods and tools for description and analysis (absolute numbers, relative differences, odd ratios, concentration index, regression, component analysis, descriminant analysis, ...). The following abstracts are examples of papers which dealt recently with this topic.

Naturally, the straightway to study health inequalities is to measure absolute and/or relative differences [21-28]

Pamuk ER. Social class inequality in mortality from 1921 to 1972 in England and Wales. Population Studies 1985; 39:17-31

Pamuk ER. Social class inequality in infant mortality in England and Wales from 1921 to 1980. Europ J Population 1988; 4:1-21

Plotting the data and fitting a regression line (y= $\square$ + $\square$ x) by least squares, certain authors have used this method to define the relative index of inequality [21-29]. Pamuk used weighted least squares with weights proportional to the population size of each category and defined the relative index of inequality as: RII= $\text{-}\square$ /$\bar{y}$ where $\bar{y}$ is the overall mean death rate (note $\square$ that is negative and $\bar{y}$-$\square$ $\square$ $\square$$x$) [21,22].

Kunst AE, Mackenbach JP. Measuring socio-economic inequalities in health. Copenhagen World Health Organization 1995.

Mackenbach JP, Kunst AE. Measuring the magnitude of socio-economic inequalities in health: an overview of available measures illustrated with two examples from Europe. Soc Sci Med 1997; 44:757-771

Considering the same equations given by regression and least squares, Kunst and Mackenbach used ordinary least squares without weights and proposed a modified index given by: RII$_{KM}$ = $\tilde{\square}$ $\square$ $\square$$\square$$\bar{y}$-$\square$$x$) [23,24].

The modified index RII$_{KM}$ appears as the ratio of the mortality of the most disadvantaged (x=0) to the most advantaged (x=1) with the precision that the extreme values x = 0 and 1 do not correspond to the lowest and highest categories. This index is easily interpreted since, for instance, a value RII$_{KM}$ =2 indicates that the mortality rate of the most disadvantaged is twice as high as that of the most advantaged.

Gakidou EE, Murray CJL, Frenk J. Defining and measuring health inequality: an approach based on the distribution of health expectancy. Bull World Health Organ 2000; 78:42-54

This paper proposes an approach to conceptualizing and operationalizing the measurement of health inequality, defined as differences in health across individuals in the population. The authors define the individual mean difference (IMD ($\square$, $\square$) which compares each individual's health to the mean of the population and allows also to compare each individual's health to every other individual's health. The authors indicate that their indicator coincides with the variance when $\square$ = 2 and $\square$$\tilde{\square}$ and with the coefficient of variation when $\square$ = 2 and $\square$$\square$$_1$but $\square$ could be any value between 0 and 1 reflecting some mix of concern between relative ($\square$$\square$$_1$) and absolute ($\square$ $\tilde{\square}$) individual mean difference[30].

The definition of inequity provided in the World Health Report 2000 was mainly based on this individual approach and we will see that many authors criticized it [31]

Starfield B. Improving equity in health: A research agenda. Int J Health Services 2001; 31(3):545-566

In this paper, equity in health is defined as "the absence of systematic and potentially remediable differences in one or more aspects of health status across socially, demographically, or geographically defined populations or population subgroups". The author also defines horizontal equity as equal access to health services for equal health needs, and vertical equity, meaning that greater health services are offered to people more in need. More globally, the author discusses pathways and social determinants underlying in(equity) and proposes a research agenda on equity in health [32].

Ruth FG Williams, DP Doessel. Measuring inequality: tools and an illustration. Int J Equity Health 2006 [http://www.equityhealthj.com/content/5/1/5]

This is an interesting pedagogic paper illustrating the problem of measuring inequality in health services. The authors presented various tools for measuring a distribution with application to data on four distributions about mental health services, indicating however, that the exercise is of broader relevance than mental health. The indicators used for comparison were the standard deviation, the coefficient of variation, the relative mean deviation and the Gini coefficient. Other, less commonly used measures also were applied, such as Theil's Index of Entropy, Atkinson's Measure. Illustration was given by the Lorenz curves [33].

Tugwell P, O'Connor A, Andersson N, Mhatre S, Kristjansson E, Jacobsen MJ et al. Reduction of inequalities in health: assessing evidence-based tools. Int J Equity Health 200 [http://www.equityhealthj.com/content/5/1/11]

Stressing that reduction of health inequalities is a focus of many national and international health organisations, this paper builds on the need for pragmatic evidence-based approaches, describing a new program that focuses upon evidence based tools, which are useful for policy initiatives that reduce inequities. Precisely, this paper was based on a presentation that was given at the "Regional Consultation on Policy Tools: Equity in Population Health Reports", held in Toronto, Canada in June 2002. Five assessment tools were presented. 1) A database of systematic reviews on the effects of educational, legal, social, and health interventions to reduce unfair inequalities is being established through the Cochrane and Campbell Collaborations. 2) Decision aids and shared decision making can be facilitated in disadvantaged groups by 'health coaches' to help people become better decision makers, negotiators, and navigators of the health system; a pilot study in Chile has provided proof of this concept. 3) The CIET Cycle: Combining adapted cluster survey techniques with qualitative methods, CIET's population based applications support evidence-based decision making at local and national levels. The CIET map generates maps directly from survey or routine institutional data, to be used as evidence-based decisions aids. Complex data can be displayed attractively, providing an important tool for studying and comparing health indicators among and between different populations. 4) The Ottawa Equity Gauge is applying the Global Equity Gauge Alliance framework to an industrialised country setting. 5) The Needs-Based Health Assessment Toolkit, established to assemble information on which clinical and health policy decisions can be based, is being expanded to ensure a focus on distribution and average health indicators. The authors conclude that evidence-based planning tools have much to offer the goal of equitable health development [34].

De Vogli R, Mistry R, Gnesotto R, Cornia GA. Has the relation between income inequality and life expectancy disappeared? Evidence from Italy and top industrialised countries. J Epidemiol Community Health 2005; 59:158-162

This paper investigated the relation between income inequality and life expectancy in Italy and across 21 wealthy countries. Using Pearson correlation coefficients and multivariate linear regression and data on income inequality measured by the Gini coefficient, life expectancy at birth, per capita income, and educational attainment, the authors stated that the cross national analyses showed that the relation between income inequality and population health has not disappeared [35].

Gakidou E, King G. Measuring total health inequality: adding individual variation to group-level differences. Int J Equity Health 2002 [http://www.equityhealthj.com/content/1/1/3]

Stressing that studies have revealed large variations in average health status across social, economic, and other groups. The authors state that "no study exists on the distribution of the risk of ill-health across individuals, either within groups or across all people in a society, and as such a crucial piece of total health inequality has been overlooked. Some of the reason for this neglect has been that the risk of death, which forms the basis for most measures, is impossible to observe directly and difficult to estimate". Consequently, a measure of total health inequality was developed in this paper. According to the authors, by adapting a beta-binomial, the proposed measure encompasses all inequalities among people in a society, including variation between and within groups. The method was applied to children under age two in 50 low- and middle-income countries. The authors stated that countries with similar average child mortality differ considerably in total health inequality. Liberia and Mozambique have the largest inequalities in child survival, while Colombia, the Philippines and Kazakhstan have the lowest levels among the countries measured [36].

Scott V, Stern R, Sanders D, Reagon G, Mathews V. Research to action to address inequities: the experience of the Cape Town Equity Gauge. Int J Equity Health 2008. [http://www.equityhealthj.com/content/7/1/6]

Underlining the recognition of the importance of promoting equity to achieve health along with a global continuous increasing gap between and within countries. the paper suggests a description that looks at how the Cape Town Equity Gauge initiative, part of the Global Equity Gauge Alliance (GEGA) was endeavouring to tackle this problem. Adopting a participatory approach, both quantitative and qualitative methods were used. The studies demonstrate the value of adopting the GEGA approach of research to action, adopting three pillars of assessment and monitoring; advocacy; and community empowerment [37].

Signal L, Martin J, Reid P, Carroll C, Howden-Chapman P et al. Tackling health inequalities: moving theory to action. Int J Equity Health 2007. [http://www.equityhealthj.com/content/6/1/12]

This paper reports on health inequalities awareness-raising workshops conducted with senior New Zealand health sector staff as part of the Government's goal of reducing inequalities in health, education, employment and housing. The authors use locally adapted equity tools, requiring participants to develop action plans, and using a case study to focus discussion, were important to the success for the training. Using institutional theory was helpful in analysing how drivers of inequalities, such as racism, are built into health institutions. This New Zealand experience provides a model that may be applicable in other jurisdictions [38].

Mackenbach JP, Stirbu I, Roskam AJR, Schaap MM, Menvielle G, Leinsalu M et al, for the European Union Working Group on Socioeconomic Inequalities in Health. Socioeconomic Inequalities in Health in 22 European Countries. N Engl J Med 2008; 358:2468-81.

Using data on mortality according to education level and occupational class from census-based mortality studies, this paper compared the magnitude of inequalities in mortality and self-assessed health among 22 countries in all parts of Europe. Deaths were classified according to cause, including common causes, such as cardiovascular disease and cancer; causes related to smoking; causes related to alcohol use; and causes amenable to medical intervention, such as tuberculosis and hypertension. Measuring the association between socio-economic status and health outcomes with the tools of regression-based inequality indexes, the authors found that, in almost all countries, the rates of death and poorer self-assessments of health were substantially higher in groups of lower socioeconomic status, but the magnitude of the inequalities between groups of higher and lower socioeconomic status was much larger in some countries than in others. In conclusion, the paper stresses that inequalities might be reduced by improving educational opportunities, income distribution, health-related behaviour, or access to health care [39].

Gwatkin DR. Health inequalities and health of the poor: What do we know? What can we do? Bull World Health Organ 2000; 78:3-17

This critical reflection is part of a theme section devoted by the Bulletin of the World Health Organization to "Inequalities in health". It contributes to the discussion on action needed by proposing two initial steps for action. The first step directed towards professionals who give very high priority to the distinct but related objectives of poverty alleviation, inequality reduction, and equity enhancement. The second step requires that health policy goals, currently expressed as societal averages, be reformulated so that they point specifically to conditions among the poor and to poor-rich differences. The author suggests, for example, to take infant mortality rates among the poor or the differences in infant mortality between rich and poor sectors as indicator instead of the average infant mortality rate for the whole population [11].

Wagstaff A. Poverty and health sector inequalities. Bull World Health Organ 2002; 80:97-105

Stating that poor countries tend to have worse health outcomes than better-off countries, and within countries, poor people have worse health outcomes than better-off people, this paper shows that the association between poverty and ill-health reflects causality running in both directions. On the one side, poverty breeds ill-health, and on the other side ill-health keeps poor people poor. The author discusses evidence on inequalities in health between the poor and non-poor, and the consequences for impoverishment and income inequality associated with health care expenses. He gives an outline of what is known about the causes of inequalities and about the effectiveness of policies intended to combat them, arguing that too little is known about the impacts of such policies [12].

Wagstaff A. Socioeconomic inequalities in child mortality: comparisons across nine developing countries. Bull World Health Organ 2000; 78:19-29

Using data from the Living Standards Measurement Study and the Cebu Longitudinal Health and Nutrition Survey, this paper generates and analyses survey data on inequalities among infants and children under five years by consumption in Brazil, Cote d'Ivoire, Ghana, Nepal, Nicaragua, Pakistan, the Philippines, South Africa, and Viet Nam. Mortality distributions were compared between countries by means of concentration curves and concentration indices. The author concludes that application of concentration curves and indices showed that inequalities in infant and under five mortality were to the disadvantage of the worse-off, with statistical significance in the most part [15].

2.2 Globalisation and equity

Schuftan C. Poverty and Inequity in the Era of Globalization: Our Need to Change and to Re-conceptualize Int J Equity Health 2002 [http://www.equityhealthj.com/content/2/1/4]

In this interesting commentary, the author calls for the need to change and to re-conceptualize notions of poverty and inequity in the era of globalization. Stressing that equal relations between unequals simply reinforce inequality and that under globalization, Capitalism is creating wealth for the few and depressing local wages and conditions of employment for the many [40].

Heggenhougen HK. The epidemiology of inequity: Will research make a difference? Norsk Epidemiologi 2005; 15: 127-132

Discussing globalization and its consequences, the author enumerates positive and negative outputs. Indicating that tremendous benefits have been obtained by vast numbers of people within and between countries, citing examples of life expectancies, decline of infant mortality and millions who now have clean water and who did not have it only few years ago. On the other hand, more and more voices express that the world really is not the mutually supportive home we would like it to be. The author also calls for distinction between inequality and inequity, putting it in a matter of social justice. Interestingly, the epidemiology of poverty and inequity was illustrated through some figures such as:

1) The proportion of income in the hands of the poorest 20% of the world's population dropped from 2.3% in 1960 to 1.2% in 1998 while the richest 20% rose from 70.2% to 89% which means that the richest 20% consume 160 times that of the poorest 20%.

2) At least one fifth of the world's population (1.2 billion) live in absolute poverty, surviving with less than one US1$ a day and 3 billion survive on US2$ in what it called "moderate poverty". 3) The contrast between a 85 years female life expectancy in Japan and 36 years in Sierra Leone. 4) An estimated 100 million street children and according to the 2001 Human Development Report 24 000 people starve to death every day. 5) The author attracts attention on the fact that the largest worldwide economic enterprise, by far, is the selling of arms, 85% of which is done by the five permanent members of the UN Security Council. 6) Worldwide, only 10% of all resources for health research are spent on diseases that account for 90% of the total global disease burden, a phenomenon called by the Global Forum for Health Research: the 10/90 problem [41].

2.3 Regional level

Reidpath D, Allotey P. Measuring global health inequity. Int J Equity Health 2007 [http://www.equityhealthj.com/content/6/1/16]

Using global health data from the World Health Organization's 14 mortality sub-regions, a measure of global health inequality (based on a decomposition of the Pietra Ratio) was contrasted with a new measure of global health inequity. Indicating that global health inequality do not take account of the health inequity associated with the additional, and unfair, encumbrances that poor health status confers on economically deprived populations, the authors made an interesting point by considering the inequality data by regional economic capacity (GNP per capita). They found that the least healthy global sub-region is shown to be around four times worse off under a health inequity analysis than would be revealed under a straight health inequality analysis. In contrast the healthiest sub-region is shown to be about four times better off. The inequity of poor health experienced by poorer regions around the world is significantly worse than a simple analysis of health inequality reveals [42].

Gwatkin D. The need for equity-oriented health sector reforms. Int J Epidemiology 2001; 30:720-723

In the six African countries considered, recent data show that income or consumption in the top 20% of the population is from five to twenty times as high as in the poorest 20%. Yet, the government health service expenditures generally reinforce rather than counterbalance those income/consumption inequalities. According to the author, the government expenditures tend to benefit Africa's richest people more than its poorest in absolute terms. On average, the highest 20% of the population receives well over twice as much financial benefit as the lowest 20% from overall government health service spending (30% *versus* 12% of total benefit)[43]

2.4 National level

In this subsection, we relate papers which have dealt with different aspects of health equity in different countries.

Low A, Ithindi T, Low A. A step too far? Making health equity interventions in Namibia more sufficient. Int J Equity Health 2003. [http://www.equityhealthj.com/content/2/1/5]

The authors have formulated a framework for relating health equity goals to development strategies allowing progressive redistribution of primary health care resources towards the more deprived communities. The framework was then applied to the development of primary health care in post-independence Namibia.

The authors conclude that the goal of equality of health status may not be appropriate in many developing country situations. They further indicate that a stepwise approach based on progressive redistribution of medical services and resources may be more appropriate. Such a conclusion challenges the views of health economists who emphasise the need to select a single health equality goal and of development agencies which stress that equality of health status is the most important dimension of health equity [44].

Van de Poel E, Hosseinpoor AR, Jehu-Appiah C, Vega J, Speybroeck N. Malnutrition and the disproportional burden on the poor: the case of Ghana. Int J Equity Health 2007 [http://www.equityhealthj.com/content/6/1/21]

Using data from the Ghana 2003 Demographic and Health and stressing that malnutrition is a major public health and development concern in the developing world and in poor communities within these regions, this paper uses a concentration index to summarize inequality in children's height-for age z-scores in Ghana across the entire socioeconomic distribution and decomposes this inequality into different contributing factors. The authors conclude that child malnutrition in Ghana is a multi-sectoral problem. The factors associated with average malnutrition rates are not necessarily the same as those associated with socioeconomic inequality in malnutrition. Not surprisingly, malnutrition was seen to be related to poverty, maternal education, health care and family planning and regional characteristics [45].

Zere E, Mandlhate C, Mbeeli T, Shangula K, Mutirua K, Kapenambili W. Equity in health care in Namibia: developing a needs-based resource allocation formula using principal components analysis. Int J Equity Health 2007 [http://www.equityhealthj.com/content/6/1/3]

Using data from the Namibia Demographic and Health Survey of 2000, the authors employed Principal components analysis to compute asset indices from asset based and health-related variables. The asset indices then formed the basis of proposals for regional weights for establishing a needs based resource allocation formula. Comparing the current allocations of public sector health car resources with estimates using a needs based formula showed that regions with higher levels of need currently receive fewer resources than do regions with lower needs. The paper concludes that to address the prevailing inequities in resource allocation, the Ministry of Health and Social Services should abandon the historical incrementalist method of budgeting/resource allocation and adopt a more appropriate allocation mechanism that incorporates measures of need for health care [46].

Yiengprugsawan V, Lim LLY, Carmichael GA, Sidorenko A, Sleigh AC. Measuring and decomposing inequity in self-reported morbidity and self-assessed health in Thailand. Int J Equity Health 2007 [http://www.equityhealthj.com/content/6/1/23]

Based on the Health and Welfare Survey 2003 conducted in Thailand by the Thai National Statistical Office with 37,202 adult respondents, an analysis was carried out in this paper. The findings confirm that substantial socioeconomic inequalities in health as measured by self-reported morbidity and self-assessed health exist in Thailand. Decomposition analysis shows that inequalities in health status are associated with particular demographic, socioeconomic and geographic population subgroups. Vulnerable subgroups which are prone to both ill health and relative poverty warrant targeted policy attention [47].

Mackenbach JP, Stronks K. The development of a strategy for tackling health inequalities in the Netherlands. Int J Equity Health 2007 [http://www.equityhealthj.com/content/3/1/11]

Reporting on the development of a strategy to reduce health inequalities in the Netherlands by an independent committee, the paper indicates that a 6-year research and development program was conducted which covered a number of different policy options and consisted of 12 intervention studies. According to the authors, although the Dutch approach has been influenced by similar efforts in other European countries, particularly the United Kingdom and Sweden, it is unique in terms of its emphasis on building a systematic evidence-base for interventions and policies to reduce health inequalities. Both researchers and policy-makers were involved in the process, and there are clear indications that some of the recommendations are being adopted by health policy-makers and health care practice, although more so at the local than at the national level [48]

Garenne M, Hohmann-Garenne S. A Wealth Index to Screen High-risk Families: Application to Morocco. J Health Popul Nutr 2003; 21: 235-242

This study analysed data collected in Morocco via the 1992 Demographic Health Survey. The author proposed a single score based on 15 socio-economic indicators as a discriminatory tool for screening families at high-risk of infant and child mortality. The wealth index defined was seen to be strongly correlated with the survival of children aged less than five years [49].

3. SOCIAL DETERMINANTS OF HEALTH

As stated by the WHO Commission on the Social Determinants of Health, in countries at all levels of income, health and illness follow a social gradient: the lower the socioeconomic position, the worse the health [3]. This statement implies that health in(equity) results from the conditions in which people are born, grow, work and age. It indicates clearly the importance of socio-economic conditions or what is now commonly known as social determinants of health, including, but not limited to factors such as food security, safe water, sanitation, education, housing and working conditions. Under this section, we summarise contributions devoted to social determinants of health at regional and national levels.

Marmot M, Friel S. Global health equity: evidence for action on the social determinants of health. J Epidemiol Community Health 2008; 62:1095-1097

In line with the report of the WHO commission on social determinants of health, this paper discusses what constitutes evidence for action. The authors recall that two headlines captured attention when the report was published. The first was the contrast between life expectancy of 43 for a woman in Zambia compared with 86 for a woman in Japan. The second was the 28 years life expectancy gap between men in Calton in Glascow and men in Lenzie 13 km away. While stressing the difficulty and difference of getting evidence from analytical studies and randomised controlled trials, the authors describe the social determinants of health as the circumstances in which people are born, grow, live, work and age; and the inequitable distribution of power, money and resources that are drivers of those circumstances of daily life [50,51].

Watts S, Siddiqi S. Social Determinants of Health in the Eastern Mediterranean Region: A discussion paper. Division of Health Systems and Services Development WHO, EMRO 2006.

Stressing that WHO Eastern Mediterranean Regional Office has been advocating poverty reduction as a strategy to facilitate equitable health development through Community Based initiatives, and expressing the multidimensional and interrelated aspects of social determinants of health, this report is gives an interesting coverage of the social determinants underlying health inequalities in the Eastern Mediterranean Region. From Morocco to Pakistan, differences are considered between and within countries and inequalities are illustrated in terms of income, average health indicators, access to health services, legislations, rural-urban, gender, migrants and others. The social determinants identified by the authors as being of regional importance include: Women's empowerment, child labour and street children and their health, migrant workers, inequitable health systems, socially determined lifestyles and behaviours, health inequities dues to conflicts. The strategies proposed for addressing the SDH in the region include: development of a solid evidence base; inclusion of SDH in national policies and programs; development of partnerships and enhancement of Community Based Initiatives [52].

Schofield T. Health inequity and its social determinants: A sociological commentary. Health Sociology Review 2007; 16(2):105-114

Suggesting that advancing efficacious policy interventions in the field of health and equity can be offered by a more dynamic understanding of the social, as provided by critical sociology, this paper explores the fundamental goals, principles and concepts of the health equity 'movement', and its relationship to the 'social determinants of health' approach. The author argues that such an approach is an instrument for rendering the problem of health inequity real and actionable by institutional authorities and policy practitioners [53].

Tugwell P, Petticrew M, Robinson V, Kristjansson E, Maxwell L, for the Cochrane Equity Field Editorial Team. Cochrane and Campbell Collaborations, and health equity. Lancet 2006; 367:1128-1130

Stressing that despite gains in average population health throughout the world, important disparities remain, this paper indicates that average goals like the Millennium Development targets can be achieved without any improvement in health and development of poor populations. The authors give examples showing how average mortality ratios conceal meaningful differences between poor and rich populations. For instance, in Peru the mean IMR is 49.9, IMR in poor is 78.3 and IMR in rich is 19.5; and in Mozambique the ratios are respectively 147.4, 187.7 and 94.7. The authors also provide an analytical framework for assessment of equity-relevant differences in intervention effectiveness, including place of residence; race, ethnic origin and culture; occupation; gender; religion; education; socio-economic status and social capital [54].

Kunst AE, Bos V, Lahelma E, Bartley M, Lissau I, Regidor E et al. Trends in socioeconomic inequalities in self-assessed health in 10 European countries. Int J Epidemiology 2005; 34(2):295-305

In this study, data were obtained from nationally representative interview surveys held in Finland, Sweden, Norway, Denmark, England, The Netherlands, West Germany, Austria, Italy, and Spain. The main objective was to determine whether inequalities in self-assessed health in the 10 European countries showed a general tendency either to increase or to decrease between the 1980s and the 1990s and whether trends varied among countries. The authors found that "socioeconomic inequalities in self-assessed health showed a high degree of stability in European countries. For all countries together, the odds ratios (ORs) comparing low with high educational levels remained stable for men (2.61 in the 1980s and 2.54 in the 1990s) but increased slightly for women (from 2.48 to 2.70). The ORs comparing extreme income quintiles increased from 3.13 to 3.37 for men and from 2.43 to 2.86 for women. Increases could be demonstrated most clearly for Italian and Spanish men and women, and for Dutch women, whereas inequalities in health in the Nordic countries showed no tendency to increase". The paper concludes: "the results underscore the persistent nature of socioeconomic inequalities in health in modern societies. The relatively favourable trends in the Nordic countries suggest that these countries' welfare states were able to buffer many of the adverse effects of economic crises on the health of disadvantaged groups" [55].

van Lenthe FJ, Borrell LN, Costa G, Roux AVD, Kauppinen TM, Marinacci C et al. Neighbourhood unemployement and all cause mortalmity: a comparison of six countries. J Epiemiol Community Health 2005; 56: 231-237

This paper was based on data from three prospective cohort studies (ARIC(US), GLOBE(Netherldans), and Whithall II (England)) and three population based register studies (Helsinki, Turin, Madrid). Cox proportional hazards models were used to assess the associations between neighbourhood unemployment and all cause mortality, adjusted for education and occupation at the individual level. The authors concluded that living in more deprived neighbourhoods is associated with increased all cause mortality in the US and five European countries, independently of individual socio-economic characteristics [56].

Merlo J, Gerdtham UG, Lynch J, Beckman1 A, Norlund A, Lithman T. Social inequalities in health- do they diminish with age? Revisiting the question in Sweden 1999. Int J Equity Health 200 [http://www.equityhealthj.com/content 2/1/2]

This study is based on an age stratified cross-sectional analysis using averages, logistic and linear regression modelling of health care contacts, health care expenditures and mortality in relation to individual income in five groups by quintiles. The population consisted of all the 249,855 men aged 40 to 80 years living in the county of Skåne, Sweden during 1999. The authors found that for working-age people (40-59 year old) a clear socio-economic gradient with increasing probability of health care contact, relative expenditure and mortality as income decreased. Estimations were given for 1st (highest)-2nd-3rd-4th and 5th (lowest) income groups and for health care contact, relative expenditure and mortality respectively. The elderly (75-80 year old) was also considered. The paper concludes, as expected among working-age individuals, lower income was associated with higher health care contact, relative expenditure and mortality. However, the existence of opposite socioeconomic gradients in health care utilisation and mortality in the elderly suggests that factors related to a high income might condition allocation of resources, or that current medical care is ineffective to treat determinants of income differences in mortality occurring earlier in the life course [57].

Boutayeb A. Social inequalities and health inequity in Morocco. Int J Equity Health 2006 [http://www.equityhealthj.com/content 5//1/1]

Recalling that despite the progress made in controlling preventable diseases, social inequalities and health inequities remain the major problems for the third millennium, this paper illustrates gaps and inequalities between urban and rural areas; poor and rich families; and developed and deprived regions in Morocco. The author gives a multitude of indicators showing unjustifiable and unfair inequalities either between different socio-economic groups or between different regions [58].

Valle AM. Social class, marginality and self-assessed health: a cross-sectional analysis of the health gradient in Mexico. Int J Equity Health 2009 [http://www.equityhealthj.com/content/8/1/3]

Using individual level data from the Second National Health Survey (ENSA II), social class categories were specified following a stratification approach according to the occupation and education indicators available from ENSA II, then authors made two types of categories, one for the urban and one for the rural labour force. Two indicators of perceived health status were used as health outcomes: self-assessed health and reported morbidity.

Furthermore, the marginality index, an indicator of relative deprivation was used to examine its contextual effect at the state and regional level. In order to examine the gradient effect of social class, logistic multivariate models were used. According to the authors, the findings of this study provided empirical evidence that social inequality negatively influences health through a differential exposure and an unequal distribution of resources across the class spectrum: the lower the social class, the poorer the perception of health. The results also showed that living in more deprived regions had a further negative effect on health [59].

Other papers were dedicated to social determinants and health equity [60-64].

4. DISEASES & EQUITY

This section is devoted to papers dealing with equity and different illnesses, including non communicable diseases in developing countries [65], neglected diseases in developing countries [66], AIDS and HIV [67,68], Malaria in Malawi and Nigeria [69,70], Tuberculosis in Malawi [71], different sites of cancer in Spain and Brazil [72,73] and depression [74,75].

Boutayeb A, Boutayeb S. The burden of non communicable diseases in developing countries. Int J Equity Health 2005 [http://www.equityhealthj.com/content/4/1/2]

Stressing that by the dawn of the third millennium, non communicable diseases (NCDS) are sweeping the whole globe, with an increasing trend in developing countries where, the transition imposes more constraints to deal with the double burden of infective and non-infective diseases in a poor environment characterised by ill-health systems, this paper gives an exhaustive overview of the non communicable diseases burden in developing countries. The authors pointed out the fact that the costly prolonged treatment of NCDs raises the equity problem between and within countries. In low- and middle-income countries, the scarce family and societal resources are often diverted to cover treatment and care and consequently, the lower socio-economic groups will have greater prevalence of risk factors, higher incidence of diseases and higher mortality [65].

Boutayeb A. Developing countries and neglected diseases: challenges and perspectives. Intern J Eq Health 2007 [http://www.equityhealthj.com/content/6/1/20]

Recalling that, despite their low mortality, neglected diseases are causing severe and permanent disabilities and deformities affecting approximately 1 billion people in the world, yielding more than 20 million of Disability Adjusted Life Years and important socio-economic losses, this commentary shows that the so-called (most) neglected tropical diseases have been given little attention mainly because investing in drugs of these diseases is thought to be not marketable or profitable. The author calls for a more equitable deal with diseases affecting poorer populations living in low- and middle-income countries [66].

Essien EJ, Ross MW, Williams ML, Meshack AF, Fernández-Esquer ME, Peters RJ *et al.* Primary source of income is associated with differences in HIV risk behaviours in street-recruited samples. Int J Equity Health 2004 [http://www.equityhealthj.com/content/3/1/5]

Self-reported data on primary source of income and HIV risk behaviours were collected from 1494 African American, Hispanic, Asian, and White men and women in places of public congregation in Houston, Texas. Data were analyzed using calculation of percentages and by chi-square tests with Yates correction for discontinuity where appropriate. According to the authors, a higher proportion of whites were involved in sex for money exchanges compared to the other racial groups in this sample. The data suggest that similar street sampling approaches are likely to recruit different proportions of people by primary income source and by ethnicity. It may be that the study locations sampled are likely to preferentially attract those involved in illegal activities, specifically the white population involved in sex for drug or money exchanges. In conclusion, this paper suggests that social disadvantage is associated with HIV risk in part by its association with drug and sex work for survival, and offers one variable that may be associated with the concentration of disease among those at greatest disadvantage by having an illegal and unstable primary income source [67].

Uzochukwu BSC, Onwujekwe OE. Socio-economic differences and health seeking behaviour for the diagnosis and treatment of malaria: a case study of four local government areas operating the Bamako initiative programme in south-east Nigeria. Int J Equity Health 2004 [http://www.equityhealthj.com/content/3/1/6

Stressing that malaria is one of the leading causes of mortality and morbidity in Nigeria, this paper deals with reliable information needed to initiate new policy thrusts to protect the poor from the adverse effect of user fees introduced under the Bamako Initiative (BI) system. Using a structured questionnaire to collect information from 1594 female household primary care givers or household head on their socio-economic and demographic status and use of malaria diagnosis and treatment services. The statistical methods used were: 1) Principal components analysis to create a socio-economic status index (decomposed into quartiles) 2) Chi-square for trends was used to calculate for any statistical difference. The study showed that self diagnosis was the commonest form of diagnosis by the respondents. This was followed by diagnosis through laboratory tests, community health workers, family members and traditional healers. Self diagnosis was practiced more by the poorer households while the least poor used the patent medicine dealers and community health workers less often for diagnosis of malaria. The least poor groups had a higher probability of seeking treatment at the BI health centres (creating equity problem in BI), hospitals, and private clinics and in using laboratory procedures. The least poor also used the patent medicine dealers and community health workers less often for the treatment of malaria. The richer households complained more about poor staff attitude and lack of drugs as their reasons for not attending the BI health centres. The factors that encourage people to use services in BI health [69]

Mathanga DP, Bowie C. Malaria control in Malawi: are the poor being served? Int J Equity Health 2007 [http://www.equityhealthj.com/content/6/1/22].

In this paper, equity in access to malaria control measures was assessed using the Malawi Demographic Health Survey (DHS) 2000 and the 2004 national survey on malaria control. Utilisation of malaria control methods was compared across the wealth quintiles, to determine whether the poor were being reached with malaria control measures. The authors state that, although coverage increased from 5% in 2000 to 35% in 2004, there was a disproportionate concentration amongst the least poor compared to the poorest group. Effective treatment of fever remains unacceptably low with only 17% of the under-five children being promptly treated with an effective anti-malarial drug. And only 29% of pregnant women received the recommended dose of at least two doses during the pregnancy. No income related inequalities were associated with prompt treatment and intermittent preventive treatment (IPT) use. The authors conclude that the present distribution strategies for insecticide-treated nets (ITNs) are not addressing the needs of the vulnerable groups, especially the poor. Increasing access to ITNs by the poor will require innovative distribution models which deliberately target the poorest of the poor [70].

Simwaka BN, Bello G, Banda H, Chimzizi R, Squire BSB, Theobald SJ. The Malawi National Tuberculosis Programme: an equity analysis. Int J Equity Health 2007 [http://www.equityhealthj.com/content/6/1/24]

Indicating that until 2005, the Malawi National Tuberculosis Control Programme had been implemented as a vertical programme. Working within the Sector Wide Approach (SWAp) provides a new environment and new opportunities for monitoring the equity performance of the programme. This paper synthesizes what is known on equity and TB in Malawi and highlights areas for further action and advocacy. A synthesis of a wide range of published and unpublished reports and studies using a variety of methodological approaches was undertaken and complemented by additional analysis of routine data on access to TB services. The analysis and recommendations were developed, through consultation with key stakeholders in Malawi and a review of the international literature. According to the authors, the lack of a prevalence survey severely limits the epidemiological knowledge base on TB and vulnerability, the major challenge being to increase case detection, especially amongst the poor, where most 'missing cases' are assumed to be found. They indicate that TB cases have increased rapidly from 5,334 in 1985 to 28,000 in 2006. This increase has been attributed to HIV/AIDS; 77% of TB patients are HIV positive. The costs of seeking TB care are high for poor women and men – up to 240% of monthly income as compared to 126% of monthly income for the non-poor [70].

Antunes JLF, Carme Borrell, Pérez G, Boing AF, Wünsch-Filho V. Inequalities in mortality of men by oral and pharyngeal cancer in Barcelona, Spain and São Paulo, Brazil, 1995–2003. Int J Equity Health 2008 [http://www.equityhealthj.com/content/7/1/14]

This paper compares socioeconomic inequalities in male mortality by oral and pharyngeal cancer in two major cities of Europe and South America, namely Barcelona in Spain and São Paulo in Brazil. Using f or each city, data on mortality provided by the official system of information. Age-adjusted death rates by oral and pharyngeal cancer for men were independently assessed for neighbourhoods of Barcelona, and São Paulo, from 1995 to 2003. Uniform methodological criteria instructed the comparative assessment of magnitude, trends and spatial distribution of mortality. General linear models assessed ecologic correlations between death rates and socioeconomic indices (unemployment, schooling levels and the human development index) at the inner-city area level. Results obtained for each city were subsequently compared. The results showed that mortality of men by oral and pharyngeal cancer ranked higher in Barcelona (9.45 yearly deaths per 100,000 male inhabitants) than in Spain and Europe as a whole; rates were on decrease. São Paulo presented a poorer profile, with higher magnitude (11.86) and stationary trend. The appraisal of ecologic correlations indicated an unequal and inequitably distributed burden of disease in both cities, with poorer areas tending to present higher mortality. Barcelona had a larger gradient of mortality than São Paulo, indicating a higher inequality of cancer deaths across its neighbourhoods [71].

Goyder E, Dibben C, Grimsley M, Peters J, Blank L, Ellis E. Variation in prescribing for anxiety and depression: a reflection of health inequalities, cultural differences or variations in access to care? Int J Equity Health 2006[http://www.equityhealthj.com/content/6/1/21]

Stating that equitable financing is a key objective of health care systems, the primary purpose of this study was to comprehensively assess the equity of health care financing in Malaysia. The paper evaluated each of the five financing sources (direct taxes, indirect taxes, contributions to Employee Provident Fund and Social Security Organization, private insurance and out-of-pocket payments). The method used was cross-sectional analyses performed on the Household Expenditure Survey Malaysia 1998/99, using Stata statistical software package and Kakwani's progressivity index. Results showed that Malaysia's predominantly tax-financed system was slightly progressive with a Kakwani's progressivity index of 0.186. The net progressive effect was produced by four progressive finance sources (in the decreasing order of direct taxes, private insurance premiums, out-of-pocket payments, contributions to EPF and SOCSO) and a regressive finance source (indirect taxes) [74].

5. CHILD HEALTH & EQUITY

The study of equity in child health is one of the most documented topics. Availability of Demographic and Health Surveys data in many developing countries allows for studies and comparisons of different health indicators in general and those measuring inequalities in particular.

Houweling TAJ, Kunst AE, Mackenbach JP. Measuring health inequality among children in developing countries: does the choice of the indicator of economic status matter? Int J Equity Health 2003 [http://www.equityhealthj.com/content/2/1/8]

Stressing that until now, there is a lack of evidence on the extent to which the use of different measures of economic status affects the observed magnitude of health inequalities, this paper provides this empirical evidence for 10 developing countries, using the Demographic and Health Surveys data-set. The authors compared the World Bank asset index to three alternative wealth indices, all based on household assets. Under-5 mortality and measles immunisation coverage were the health outcomes studied. Poor-rich inequalities in under-5 mortality and measles immunisation coverage were measured using the Relative Index of Inequality. In conclusion, attention is attracted by the fact that researchers and policy makers should be aware that the choice of the measure of economic status influences the observed magnitude of health inequalities, and that differences in health inequalities between countries or time periods, may be an artefact of different wealth measures used [76].

van de Poel E, Hosseinpoor AR, Sneybroeck N, Ourti TV, Vega J. Socioeconomic inequality in malnutrition in developing countries. Bull World Health Organ 2007; 86:282-291.

Using component analysis and a generalization of the concentration index to analyse data from 47 developing countries, this study have shown that socioeconomic inequality in malnutrition is present throughout these countries [17]. Estimating stunting and wasting rates in children aged less than five years according to socioeconomic status the authors illustrated clearly the differences between children belonging to the wealthiest quintiles compared to those from the poorest quintiles. As shown in Table 6, children from poorest [77]

Houweling TAJ, Kunst AE, Huisman M, Mackenbach JP. Using relative and absolute measures for monitoring health inequalities: experiences from cross-national analyses on maternal and child health. Int J Equity Health 2007 [http://www.equityhealthj.com/content/6/1/15]

Wealth-group specific data on under-5 mortality, immunisation coverage, antenatal and delivery were obtained from the Demographic and Health Surveys of 43 countries and used to describe the association between the overall level of these health indicators and relative and absolute poor-rich inequalities. This paper demonstrates that the values that the absolute and relative inequality measures can take are bound by mathematical ceilings. Yet, even where these ceilings do not play a role, the magnitude of inequality is correlated with the overall level of the outcome. The observed tendencies are, however, not necessities. There are countries with low mortality levels and low relative inequalities. Also absolute inequalities showed variation at most overall levels. The authors conclude that both absolute and relative inequality measures can be meaningful for monitoring inequalities, provided that the overall level of the outcome is taken into account [78]

Fotso JC. Child health inequities in developing countries: differences across urban and rural areas. Int J Equity Health 2006[http://www.equityhealthj.com/content/5/1/9]

Using the most recent data available from the DHS of 15 countries in sub-Saharan Africa (SSA), this paper considered the magnitude of inequities in child malnutrition across urban and rural areas. The findings were that "across countries in SSA, though socioeconomic inequalities in stunting do exist in both urban and rural areas, they are significantly larger in urban areas". The authors further stated that intra-urban differences in child malnutrition are larger than overall urban-rural differentials in child malnutrition, and there seem to be no visible relationships between within-urban inequities in child health on the one hand, and urban population growth, urban malnutrition, or overall rural-urban differentials in malnutrition, on the other. Finally, maternal and father's education, community SES and other measurable covariates at the mother and child levels only explain a slight part of the within-urban differences in child malnutrition. The authors conclude that the urban advantage in health masks enormous disparities between the poor and the non-poor in urban areas of SSA [79]

Khawaja M, Dawns J, Meyerson-Knox S, Yamout R. Disparities in child health in the Arab region during the 1990s. Int J Equity Health 2008 [http://www.equityhealthj.com/content/7/1/214]

In this paper, using available tabulations and reliable micro data from national household surveys, data for 18 Arab countries were analysed, focusing on infant and child mortality, nutritional status, vaccination, and Acute Respiratory Infection (ARI). Within-country disparities in child health by gender, residence (urban/rural) and maternal educational level were described. Child health was also analyzed by macro measures of development, including per capita GDP (PPP), female literacy rates, urban population and doctors per 100,000 people. Stressing that, while Arab countries showed an impressive decline in child mortality rates during the past few decades, gaps in mortality by gender and socioeconomic status persisted, the authors conclude that with the exception of infant and child survival, gender disparities demonstrated a female advantage, as well as a large urban advantage and an overall advantage for mothers with secondary education. Surprisingly, the countries' rankings with respect to disparities were not associated with various macro measures of development [80]

Chen E, Martin AD, Matthews KA. Socioeconomic status and health: Do gradients differ within childhood and adolescence. Soc Sci Med 2006; 62-2161-2170

Based on data from the National Health Interview Survey (NHIS), the authors found that, child health status differ significantly between richer and poorer households but the differences do not increase as children grow up [81]. This result is, however, contrasting with the findings of other authors using the same data source and claiming that the relationship between household income and children's health and its lasting impact as children age, with no diminution of the gradient in adolescence [82].

Zere E, McIntyre D. Inequities in under-five child malnutrition in South Africa. Int J Equity Health 2003 [http://www.equityhealthj.com/content/2/1/7]

Using data on 3765 under-five children derived from the Living Standards and Development Survey, and considering household income (per capita household expenditure as a proxy) as the main indicator of socio-economic status, the objective of this paper was to assess and quantify the magnitude of inequalities in under-five child malnutrition, particularly those ascribable to socio-economic status and to consider the policy implications of these findings. Underlining that reliance on global averages alone can be misleading, the authors conclude that: "there are significant differences in under-five child malnutrition (stunting and underweight) that favour the richest of society. These are unnecessary, avoidable and unjust. It is demonstrated that addressing such socio-economic gradients in ill-health, which perpetuate inequalities in the future adult population requires a sound evidence base" [83].

Wamani H, Tylleskär T, Åstrøm AN, Tumwine JK, Peterson S. Mothers' education but not fathers' education, household assets or land ownership is the best predictor of child health inequalities in rural Uganda. Int J Equity Health 2004 [http://www.equityhealthj.com/content/3/1/9

Stressing that health and nutrition inequality is a result of a complex web of factors that include socio-economic inequalities, the objective of this paper was to examine the association of four socio-economic indicators namely: mothers' education, fathers' education, household asset index, and land ownership with growth stunting, which was used as a proxy for health and nutrition inequalities among infants and young children. The authors stated that various socio-economic indicators exist however some do not accurately predict inequalities in children while others are not intervention feasible. Consequently this paper was based on a cross-sectional survey conducted in the rural district of Hoima, Uganda, using two-stage cluster sampling design to obtain 720 child/mother pairs. In order to gather information on indicators of household socio-economic status and child anthropometry, a structured questionnaire was addressed to mothers in their home settings then a Regression modelling was used to determine the association of socio-economic indicators with stunting. The results showed that 25% of the studied children were stunted, of which 61% were boys. Analysis also indicated a higher prevalence of stunting among children of: non-educated mothers compared to mothers educated above primary school; non-educated fathers compared to fathers educated above secondary school; households belonging in the "poorest" quintile for the asset index compared to the "least poor" quintile; Land ownership exhibited no differentials with stunting. Finally, adjusting all socio-economic indicators in conditional regression analysis left mothers' education as the only independent predictor of stunting with children of non-educated mothers significantly more likely to be stunted compared to those of mothers educated above primary school [84].

Hong R, Banta JE, Betancourt JA. Relationship between household wealth inequality and chronic childhood under-nutrition in Bangladesh. Int J Equity Health 20006[http://www.equityhealthj.com/content/5/1/15]

Using information from 5,977 children aged 0-59 months included in the 2004 Bangladesh Demographic and Health Survey, this study examined the relationship between household wealth inequality and chronic childhood under-nutrition. The paper confirms the poor-rich inequity existing in child health. Indeed, the results indicate that children in the poorest 20% of households are more than three time as likely to suffer from adverse growth rate stunting as children from the wealthiest 20% of households. Moreover, the effect of household wealth status remain significantly large when the analysis was adjusted for a child's multiple birth status, age, gender, antenatal care, delivery assistance, birth order, and duration that the child was breastfed; mother's age at childbirth, nutritional status, education; household access to safe drinking water, arsenic in drinking water, access to a hygienic toilet facility, cooking fuel cleanliness, residence, and geographic location. The study concludes that household wealth inequality is strongly associated with childhood adverse growth rate stunting. Reducing poverty and making services more available and accessible to the poor are essential to improving overall childhood health and nutritional status in Bangladesh [85].

Razzaque A, Streatfield PK, Gwatkin DR. Does health intervention improve socioeconomic inequalities of neonatal, infant and child mortality? Evidence from Matlab, Bangladesh. Int J Equity Health 2007 [http://www.equityhealthj.com/content/6/1/4]

The findings of this paper were based on four birth cohorts (1983–85, 1988–90, 1993–95, 1998–00) followed for five years for death and out-migration in two adjacent areas (ICDDR,B-service and government-service) with similar socioeconomic but different health services. Based on asset quintiles, inequality was measured through both poor-rich ratio and concentration index. The study found that the socioeconomic inequalities of neonatal, infant and under-five mortality increased over time in both the ICDDR,B-service and government-service areas but it declined substantially for 1–4 years in the ICDDR,B- service area. The study concluded that usual health intervention programs (non-targeted) do not reduce poor-rich gap, rather the gap increases initially but might decrease in long run if the program is very intensive[86].

Giashuddin SM, Rahman A, Rahman F, Mashrekey SR, Chowdhury SM, Linnan M et al. Socioeconomic inequality in child injury in Bangladesh - implication for developing countries. Int J Equity Health 2009 [http://www.equityhealthj.com/content/8/1/7]

This study was based on data from Bangladesh Health and Injury Survey for 1-4 years children, using a multistage cluster sampling technique and considering quintiles of socioeconomic status calculated on the basis of assets and wealth score obtained by principle component analysis. The numerical measures of inequality in mortality and morbidity were assessed by the concentration index. The findings are that "the poorest-richest quintile ratio of mortality due to injury was 6.0 whereas this ratio was 5.6 and 5.5 for the infectious diseases and non-communicable diseases. The values of mortality concentration indices for child mortality due to infection, non-communicable diseases and injury causes were -0.40, -0.32 and -0.26 respectively. Among the morbidity concentration indices, injury showed significantly greater inequality. All the concentration indices revealed that there were significant inequalities among the groups. The logistic regression analysis indicated that poor children were 2.8 times more likely to suffer from injury mortality than rich children, taking into account all the other factors"[87].

Khun S, Manderson L. Poverty, user fees and ability to pay for health care for children with suspected dengue in rural Cambodia. Int J Equity Health 2008 [http://www.equityhealthj.com/content/7/1/10]

User fees were introduced in public health facilities in Cambodia in 1997 in order to inject funds into the health system to enhance the quality of services. Because of inadequate health insurance, a social safety net scheme was introduced to ensure that all people were able to attend the health facilities. However, continuing high rates of hospitalization and mortality from dengue fever among infants and children reflect the difficulties that women continue to face in finding sufficient cash in cases of medical emergency, resulting in delays in diagnosis and treatment. In this article, drawing on in-depth interviews conducted with mothers of children infected with dengue in eastern Cambodia, the authors illustrate the profound economic consequences for households when a child is ill. The direct costs for health care and medical services, and added indirect costs, deterred poor women from presenting with sick children. Those who eventually sought care often had to finance health spending through out-of-pocket payments and loans, or sold property, goods or labour to meet the costs. Costs were often catastrophic, exacerbating the extreme poverty of those least able to afford it [88].

Zhu JM, Zhu Y, Liu R Health insurance of rural/township schoolchildren in Pinggu, Beijing: coverage rate, determinants, disparities, and sustainability. Int J Equity Health 2008 [http://www.equityhealthj.com/content/7/1/23]

Based on a survey of elementary school students conducted in Pinggu, a rural/suburban district of Beijing, this paper reports findings on schoolchildren's insurance coverage, disparities between farmer and non farmer households, and effects of low-premium cooperative schemes on healthcare access and utilization. It also discusses barriers to sustainable enrolment and program growth. In order to to examine various aspects of health insurance, the authors used statistical analyses of association and adjusted odds ratio via logistic regression. They found that: "children's health insurance coverage rose to 54% by 2005, the rates are comparable for farmers' and non-farmer's children. However, 76% of insured farmers' children were covered under a low-premium scheme protecting only major medical events, compared to 42% among insured non-farmers' children. The low-premium schemes improved parental perceptions of children's access to and affordability of healthcare, their healthcare-seeking behaviours, and overall satisfaction with healthcare, but had little impact on utilization of outpatient care" [89].

6. MATERNAL HEALTH, VIOLENCE, AND HEALTH EQUITY

An important literature is being devoted to health equity in relation with maternal health [90,98].

Say L, Raine R. A systematic review of inequalities in the use of maternal health care in developing countries: examining the scale of the problem and the importance of context. Bull World Health Organ 2007; 85(10):812-819

Recalling that two decades after the Safe Motherhood campaign's launched in1987, half a million women continue to die from pregnancy-related causes every year, this paper reviewed the use of maternal health-care interventions in 23 developing countries in order to assess the extent, strength and implications of evidence of variations according to women's place of residence and socio-economic status. Thirty eligible studies were identified, of which 12 of high to moderate quality. According to the authors, this review shows variation in the use of maternal health care across populations both within and between the 23 countries considered. The paper concludes that two reasons for the limited success of the safe motherhood campaign during the last two decades have been the lack of rigorous analysis of the data available on variations in use, together with an inadequate grasp of the contextual issues that must be addressed if inequalities in maternal health care use are to be reduced. [91]

Islam M. The Safe Motherhood Initiative and beyond. Bull World Health Organ 2007; 85(10):735-735

Celebrating the 20th anniversary of the Safe Motherhood Initiative, this editorial indicates that, despite improvement of health and well-being of mothers achieved in many countries during the last two decades, globally, the numbers remain staggering: each year sees more than a half million maternal deaths, some 4 million neonatal deaths and at least 3.2 million stillborn babies of which 98% occurring in low-income countries. The author stresses the contrast between developed countries where pregnant women receive an integrated package of antenatal, childbirth and post-partum care, and developing countries where regular post-partum follow-up care is rarely available and antenatal care visits often insufficient. According to the author, the challenges to be met are not new technologies nor new knowledge about effective interventions, the real challenges are how to delivzer services and scale up interventions , particularly to those who are vulnerable, hard to reach, marginalised and excluded [92]

Houweling TAJ, Ronsmans C, Campbell OMC, Kunst AE. Huge poor-rich inequalities in maternity care: an international comparative study of maternity and child care in developing countries. Bul World Health Org. Bull World Health Org 2007; 85:745-754

Stressing that reducing poor-rich inequalities is essential to the achievement of the Millennium Development Goals (MDGs) and using Demographic Health Surveys (DHS) from 45 developing countries, this study describes poor-rich inequalities by quintiles in maternity care (professional delivery care and antenatal care), full child immunization coverage and medical treatment of diarrhoea and acute respiratory infections(ARI). The authors found that poor-rich inequalities in maternal care in general are much greater than those in immunization coverage or treatment for child illnesses. They also indicate that, although poor-rich inequalities within both rural and urban areas are large, most births without delivery assistance occur among the rural poor [93].

Collin SM, Anwar I, Ronsmans C. A decade of inequality in maternity care: antenatal care, professional attendance at delivery, and caesarean section in Bangladesh (1991–2004) Int J Equity Health 2007 [http://www.equityhealthj.com/content/6/1/9]

Recalling that Bangladesh is committed to the fifth Millennium Development Goal (MDG-5) target of reducing its maternal mortality ratio by three-quarters between 1990 and 2015. This study used data from four Demographic and Health Surveys conducted between 1993 and 2004 to examine trends in the proportions of live births preceded by antenatal consultation, attended by a health professional, and delivered by caesarean section, according to key socio-demographic characteristics. The authors found that, despite a relatively greater increase in rural than urban areas, utilization remained much lower among the poorest rural women without formal education (18%) compared with the richest urban women with secondary or higher education (99%). Professional attendance at delivery increased by 50% (from 9% to 14%, more rapidly in rural than urban areas), and caesarean sections trebled (from 2% to 6%), but these indicators remained low even by developing country standards. Within these trends there were huge inequalities; 86% of live births among the richest urban women with secondary or higher education were attended by a health professional, and 35% were delivered by caesarean section, compared with 2% and 0.1% respectively of live births among the poorest rural women without formal education [94].

Lanre-Abass BA. Poverty and maternal mortality in Nigeria: towards a more viable ethics of modern medical practice. Int J Equity Health 2008[http://www.equityhealthj.com/content/7/1/11]

Rightly underling that poverty is often identified as a major barrier to human development and is also a powerful brake on accelerated progress toward the Millennium Development Goals. The authors pointed out that poverty is also a major cause of maternal mortality, as it prevents many women from getting proper and adequate medical attention due to their inability to afford good antenatal care. The authors examine poverty as a threat for human existence and suggest ways of reducing maternal mortality in Nigeria [95].

Andersson N, Ho-Foster A.13,915 reasons for equity in sexual offences legislation: A national school-based survey in South Africa. Int J Equity Health 2008 [http://www.equityhealthj.com/content/7/1/20]

Using a facilitated self-administered questionnaire in nine of the 11 official languages in a stratified (province/metro/urban/rural) last stage random national sample, this study sought to document prevalence of male sexual violence among school-going youth. Schoolchildren answered questions about exposure in the last year to insults, beating, unwanted touching and forced sex. They indicated the sex of the perpetrator, and whether this was a family member, a fellow schoolchild, a teacher or another adult. Respondents also gave the age when they first suffered forced sex and when they first had consensual sex. The authors found that some 9% of male respondents aged 11–19 years reported forced sex in the last year. Of those aged 18 years at the time of the survey, 44% said they had been forced to have sex in their lives and 50% reported consensual sex. Perpetrators were most frequently an adult not from their own family, followed closely in frequency by other schoolchildren. Some 32% said the perpetrator was male, 41% said she was female and 27% said they had been forced to have sex by both male and female perpetrators. Male abuse of schoolboys was more common in rural areas while female perpetration was more an urban phenomenon. This study uncovers endemic sexual abuse of male children that was suspected but hitherto only poorly documented. Legal recognition of the criminality of rape of male children is a first step. The next steps include serious investment in supporting male victims of abuse, and in prevention of all childhood sexual abuse [96].

Joffres C, Mills E, Joffres M, Khanna T, Walia H, Grund D. Sexual slavery without borders: trafficking for commercial sexual exploitation in India. Int J Equity Health 2008 [http://www.equityhealthj.com/content/6/1/22]

Stressing that although trafficking in women and children is a gross violation of human rights, an estimated 800 000 women and children are trafficked each year across international borders with 80% of trafficked persons ending in forced sex work. The authors indicate that India has been identified as one of the Asian countries where trafficking for commercial sexual exploitation has reached alarming levels and that India has also emerged as an international supplier of trafficked women and children to the Gulf States and South East Asia, as well as a destination country for women and girls trafficked for commercial sexual exploitation from Nepal and Bangladesh. Pointing out also that trafficking for commercial sexual exploitation is a highly profitable and low risk business that preys on particularly vulnerable populations, this paper presents an overview of the trafficking of women and girls for sexual exploitation (CSE) in India; identifies the health impacts of CSE; and suggests strategies to respond to trafficking and related issues [97].

Demirchyan A, Thompson ME. Determinants of self-rated health in women: a population-based study in Armavir Marz, Armenia, 2001 & 2004. Int J Equity Health 2008 [http://www.equityhealthj.com/content/5/1/21]

Using data generated from cross-sectional household health surveys conducted in Armavir marz in 2001 and 2004, this study analyses differences in self-rated health in women respondents along three main dimensions: social, behavioural/attitudinal, and psychological. Overall, 2 038 women aged 18 and over participated in the two surveys (1 019 in each). The rate of perceived "poor" health was relatively high in both surveys: 38.1% in 2001 and 27.0% in 2004. The sets of independent predictors of poor self-rated health were similar in the three models considered, and included severe and moderate material deprivation, probable and possible depression, low level of education, and having ever smoked. These predictors mediated the effect of women's economic activity (including unemployment), ethnicity, low access to utilization of healthcare services, and living alone on self-rated health. The authors conclude that "Material deprivation was the most influential predictor of self-rated health. Consequently, social reforms are seen as a powerful tool for reducing health inequalities and improving the health status of the population, and hence recommended in order to decrease the gap between the rich and poor" [98].

7. GEOGRAPHIC DISPARITIES & HEALTH EQUITY

Boutayeb A, Serghini M. Health indicators and human development in the Arab Region. http://www.ij-healthgeographics.com/content/5/1/61

Using Principal Components Analysis to compare the achievements of the Arab countries in terms of direct and indirect health indicators, this paper deals with the relationship between health indicators and human development in the Arab region. The authors indicate that despite substantial economic and social progress made during the last decades by, the Arab region has accomplished less than expected in terms of human development. Huge social inequalities and health inequities exist inter and intra Arab countries. In most Arab countries, a large percentage of populations, especially in rural areas, are deprived of access to health facilities. Consequently, many women still die during pregnancy and labour, yielding unacceptable levels of maternal and infant mortality [99].

Gupta N, Zurn P, Diallo K, Dal Poz MR. Uses of population census data for monitoring geographical imbalance in the health workforce: snapshots from three developing countries. Int J Equity Health [http://www.equityhealthj.com/content/5/1/13]

In this study, population-based indicators of geographical variations among human resources for health (HRH) were extracted from census micro data samples for Kenya, Mexico and Viet Nam and health workforce statistics were matched against international standards of occupational classification to control for cross-national comparability. Summary measures of inequality were calculated to monitor the distribution of health workers across spatial units and by occupational group. Strong inequalities were found in the geographical distribution of the health workforce in all three countries, with the highest densities of HRH tending to be found in the capital areas. Cross-national differences were found in the magnitude of distributional inequality according to occupational group, with health professionals most susceptible to inequitable distribution in Kenya and Viet Nam but less so in Mexico compared to their associate professional counterparts. Some discrepancies were suggested between mappings of occupational information from the raw data with the international system, especially for nursing and midwifery specializations. The authors conclude that the problem of geographical imbalance among HRH across countries in the developing world holds important implications at the local, national and international levels, in terms of constraints for the effective deployment, management and retention of HRH, and ultimately for the equitable delivery of health services [100].

Cai L, Chongsuvivatwong V. Rural-urban differentials of premature mortality burden in south-west China. Int J Equity Health 2006 [http://www.equityhealthj.com/content/5/1/13]

This study examines the premature mortality burden from common causes of deaths among an urban region, suburban region and rural region of Kunming, the capital of Yunnan, a province located in south western China and one of the poorest provinces in the country. Years of life lost (YLL) rate per 1,000 and mortality rate per 100,000 were calculated from medical death certificates in 2003 and broken down by cause of death, age and gender among urban, suburban and rural regions. The authors found that Non-communicable diseases contributed the most YLL in all three regions. The rural region had about 50% higher premature mortality burden compared to the other two regions. YLL from infectious diseases and perinatal problems was still a major problem in the rural region. Among non-communicable diseases, YLL from stroke was the highest in the urban/suburban regions; COPD followed as the second and was the highest in the rural region. Mortality burden from injuries was however higher in the rural region than the other two regions, especially for men. Self-inflicted injuries were between 2–8 times more serious among women. The paper concludes: "the rural region is additionally burdened by diseases of poverty and injury on top of the non-communicable diseases" [101].

Kazembe LN, Appleton CC, Kleinschmidt I. Geographical disparities in core population coverage indicators for roll back malaria in Malawi. Int J Equity Health 2007 [http://www.equityhealthj.com/content/6/1/5]

Data from the 2000 Malawi Demographic and Health Survey (DHS) were aggregated at sub-district level: (1) households possessing at least one bed-net; (2) children under 5 years who slept under a bed-net the night before the survey; (3) bed-nets retreated with insecticide within past 6–12 months preceding the survey; (4) children under 5 who had fever two weeks before the survey and received treatment within 24 hours from the onset of fever;

and (5) women who received intermittent preventive treatment of malaria during their last pregnancy. Each response was geographically smoothed at sub-district level by applying conditional autoregressive models using Markov Chain Monte Carlo simulation techniques. The percentage of households possessing at least one bednet was 19%, with 9% of children sleeping under a net, while 18% of households had retreated their nets within past 12 months prior to the survey. The northern region and lakeshore areas had high bednet coverage, but low usage and re-treatment rates. Coverage rate of children who received antimalarial treatment within 24 hours after onset of fever was consistently low for most parts of the country, with mean coverage of 4.8% (95% CI: 4.5–5.0%). About 48% of women received antimalarial prophylaxis during their pregnancy, with highest rates in the southern and northern areas. The authors conclude that these results demonstrate that DHS data, with appropriate methodology, can provide acceptable estimates at sub-national level for monitoring and evaluation of malaria control goals [102].

Perry HB, King-Schultz LW, Aftab AS, Bryant JH. Health equity issues at the local level: Socio-geography, access, and health outcomes in the service area of the Hôpital Albert Schweitzer-Haiti. Int J Equity Health 2007 [http://www.equityhealthj.com/content/6/1/7]

Noting that, although health equity issues at regional, national and international levels are receiving increasing attention, health equity issues at the local level have been virtually overlooked ,this paper describes a comprehensive equity assessment carried out by the Hôpital Albert Schweitzer-Haiti (HAS) in 2003. The authors reviewed all available information arising from a comprehensive evaluation of the programs of HAS carried out in 1999 and 2000 and found markedly reduced access to health services in the peripheral mountainous areas compared to the central plains. The quality of services was more deficient and the coverage of key services was lower in the mountains. Finally, health status, as measured by under-five mortality rates and levels of childhood malnutrition, was also worse in the mountains. In conclusion, the findings indicate that local health programs need to give attention to monitoring the health status as well as the quality and coverage of basic services among marginalized groups within the program service area [103].

Ben Romdhane H, Grenier F R. Social determinants in Tunisia: the case-analysis of Ariana. Int J Equity Health 2009 [http://www.equityhealthj.com/content/8/1/9]

This strategic analysis examines selected social determinants of health in a major urban centre of Tunisia, identifies the most influential stakeholders able to influence equity/inequity, and reviews the accomplishments and need for action to foster health equity. This analysis was performed through a literature review and participatory research methods that included focus groups discussions and interview with key informants. Access to health care, changes in lifestyles, housing issues and gender-related inequities are prime, socially-determined elements that affect health in Ariana. In conclusion, recognition of emerging health issues is needed along with improved inter and intrasectoral coordination among stakeholders. The community-participatory approach used in this paper proved to be a useful scoping technique for this setting. A similar methodology could be used by other researchers as a first step toward health equity action at a city level [104].

8. MIGRANTS AND HEALTH EQUITY

Sadler GR, Ryujin L, Nguyen T, Oh G, Paik G, Kustin B. Heterogeneity within the Asian American community. Int J Equity Health 2007 [http://www.equityhealthj.com/content/2/1/12]

In this study, a convenience sample of 1,202 Asian American women evaluated the cultural alignment of a cancer education program, completing baseline and follow-up surveys that included questions about their breast cancer knowledge, attitudes, and screening behaviours. Participants took part in a brief education program that facilitated adherence to recommended screening guidelines. Statistically significant variations existed among the subgroups' breast cancer knowledge, attitudes, and screening behaviours that could contribute to health disparities among the subgroups and within the aggregate Pan Asian community. The authors conclude that health promotion efforts of providers, educators, and policy makers can be enhanced if cultural differences are identified and taken into account when developing strategies to reduce health disparities and promote health equity [105].

Ronellenfitsch U, Razum O. Deteriorating health satisfaction among immigrants from Eastern Europe to Germany. Int J Equity Health [http://www.equityhealthj.com/content/3/1/4].

Recalling that immigrants from Eastern Europe constitute more than 5% of Germany's population and their health status upon arrival may be worse than that of the native-born German population. The authors hypothesise that as a minority, they may be socio-economically disadvantaged, and their health status may deteriorate quickly. For this purpose, they compared data from 1995 and 2000 for immigrants from Eastern Europe (n = 353) and a random sample of age-matched Germans (n = 2, 824) from the German Socioeconomic Panel. We tested H1-3 using health satisfaction, as a proxy for health status, and socioeconomic indicators then compared changes over time within groups, and between immigrants and Germans. Finally they assessed effects of socio-economic status and being a migrant on declining health satisfaction in a regression model. The findings were that in 1995, immigrants under 55 years had a significantly higher health satisfaction than Germans. Above age 54, health satisfaction did not differ. By 2000, immigrants' health satisfaction had declined to German levels. Whereas in 1995 immigrants had a significantly lower SES, differences five years later had declined. In the regression model, immigrant status was much stronger associated with declining health satisfaction than low SES. In conclusion, younger immigrants had an initial health advantage. Immigrants were initially socio-economically disadvantaged but their SES improved over time. The decrease in health satisfaction was much steeper in immigrants and this was not associated with differences in SES (H3). Immigrants from Eastern Europe have a high risk of deteriorating health, in spite of socio-economic improvements [106].

Syed HR, Dalgard OS, Hussain A, Dalen I, Claussen B, Ahlberg NL. Inequalities in health: a comparative study between ethnic Norwegians and Pakistanis in Oslo, Norway. Int J Equity Health 2006 [http://www.equityhealthj.com/content/5/1/7]

The objective of the study was to observe the inequality in health from the perspective of socio-economic factors in relation to ethnic Pakistanis and ethnic Norwegians in Oslo, Norway. Data was collected by using an open and structured questionnaire, as a part of the Oslo Health Study 2000–2001. Accordingly 13581 ethnic Norwegians (45% of the eligible) participated as against 339 ethnic Pakistanis (38% of the eligible). According to the authors, the ethnic Pakistanis reported a higher prevalence of poor self-rated health 54.7% as opposed to 22.1% in ethnic Norwegians, 14% vs. 2.6% in diabetes, and 22.0% vs. 9.9% in psychological distress. The socio-economic conditions were inversely related to self- rated health, diabetes and distress for the ethnic Norwegians. However, this was surprisingly not the case for the ethnic Pakistanis. Odd ratios did not interfere with the occurrence of diabetes, even after adjusting all the markers of socio-economic status in the multivariate model, while self-reported health and distress showed moderate reduction in the risk estimation. There is a large diversity of self-related health, prevalence of diabetes and stress among the ethnic Pakistanis and Norwegians. Socio-economic status may partly explain the observed inequalities in health [107].

Bekker MHJ, Lhajoui M. Health and literacy in first- and second-generation Moroccan Berber women in the Netherlands: Ill literacy? Int J Equity Health 2004. [http://www.equityhealthj.com/content/3/1/8]

This study aimed at investigating the role of literacy and generation in the self-reported general health status of Moroccan Berber speaking women in the Netherlands. A sample of 75 women was considered, with 25 literates and 25 illiterates from the first generation, and another group of 25 literate women belonged to the second generation. The three groups were matched for demographic characteristics. According to the authors, after controlling for age, having a job, and having an employed partner, the first

generation literates compared with the illiterates of the first generation indeed reported significantly better health. Additionally, we did not find any differences in health condition between both literate groups, even after controlling for age, number of children, and marital status. Health complaints that were most frequently reported by both groups, concerned pain in shoulders, back and head. The paper concludes by underlining the importance of offering immigrants optimal access to opportunities and facilities that can improve their literacy and reading ability [108].

Kelaher M, Paul S, Lambert H, Ahmad W, Smith GD. The applicability of measures of socioeconomic position to different ethnic groups within the UK. Int J Equity Health 200[http://www.equityhealthj.com/content/8/1/4]

Based on a sample of White (n = 227), African-Caribbean (n = 213) and Indian and Pakistani (n = 233) adults aged between 18 and 59 years living in Leeds as measured in a stratified population survey, this study seeks to tease out differences in socioeconomic position between ethnic groups. According to the authors, there are 3 main reasons why conventional socioeconomic indicators and asset based measures may not be equally applicable to all ethnic groups:

1) Differences in response rate to conventional socioeconomic indicators

2) Cultural and social differences in economic priorities/opportunities

3) Differences in housing quality, assets and debt within socioeconomic strata

Measures included income, education, employment, car ownership, home ownership, housing quality, household assets, investments, debt, perceived ability to obtain various sums and perceived level of financial support given and received. The authors conclude that in the UK, education appears to be an effective variable for measuring variation in SEP across ethnic groups but the ability to account for SEP differences may be improved by the addition of car and home ownership, ability to obtain £10 000, loaning money to family/friends and income from employment/self employment. Further research is required to establish the degree to which results of this study are generalisable [109].

9. HEALTH AND EQUITY FINANCE

Yu CP, Whynes DK, Sach TH. Equity in health care financing: The case of Malaysia. Int J Equity Health 2007 [http://www.equityhealthj.com/contentent/7/1/15]

Stressing that equitable financing is a key objective of health care systems, the primary purpose of this study was to comprehensively assess the equity of health care financing in Malaysia. The paper evaluated each of the five financing sources (direct taxes, indirect taxes, contributions to Employee Provident Fund and Social Security Organization, private insurance and out-of-pocket payments), independently and subsequently by combining the financing sources to evaluate the whole financing system. Cross-sectional analyses were performed on the Household Expenditure Survey Malaysia 1998/99, using Stata statistical software package. The authors showed that Malaysia's predominantly tax-financed system was slightly progressive with a Kakwani's progressivity index of 0.186. The net progressive effect was produced by four progressive finance sources (in the decreasing order of direct taxes, private insurance premiums, out-of-pocket payments, contributions to EPF and SOCSO) and a regressive finance source (indirect taxes) [110].

Levy JI, Chemerynski SM, Tuchmann JL. Incorporating concepts of inequality and inequity into health benefits analysis. Int J Equity Health 2007

In order to develop appropriate inequality indicators for health benefits analysis, this paper provides relevant definitions from the fields of risk assessment and environmental justice and considers the implications. Axioms proposed in past studies of inequality indicators were evaluated and additional axioms relevant to this context were developed. The authors also survey the literature on previous applications of inequality indicators and evaluate five candidate indicators in reference to their proposed axioms. Finally, they present an illustrative pollution control example to determine whether their selected indicators provide interpretable information. The paper conclude that, among other, an inequality indicator for health benefits analysis should not decrease when risk is transferred from a low-risk to high-risk person, and that it should decrease when risk is transferred from a high-risk to low-risk person (Pigou-Dalton transfer principle), and that it should be able to have total inequality divided into its constituent parts (subgroup decomposability) [111].

10. MORE BIBLIOGRAPHY FOR READING

Health Sociology Review 2007; 16(2): Social Equity and Health

The World Report 2008: Primary Health Care-Now More Than Ever. Chapter I: The challenges of a changing world. Unequal growth, unequal outcomes pp2-6, Health equity p15

Sixty-second World Health Assembly resolution "Reducing health inequities through action on the social determinants of health"

11. CONFLICT INTERSET

The authors declare that they have no conflict interest

12. ACKNOWLEDGEMENTS

This paper was partly supported by a grant under the Global Project for Research (PGR) of the University Mohamed Premier, Oujda.

13. REFERENCES

1. The World Health Report 2000. Health Systems: Improving Performance. The World Health Organization, Geneva: WHO 2000
2. International Society for Equity in Health [http://www.iseqh.org/workdef_en.htm].
3. Commission on Social Determinants of health. Closing the gap in a generation: health equity through action on the social determinants of health. Geneva: World Health Organization, 2008.
4. Civil Society 2008, Social Medicine 2008, 2 (4), 192-211
5. European DETERMINE [www.health-inequalities.eu Accessed 21/7/2009]
6. The World Bank. The World Report 2006. [www.worldbank.org Accessed 21/7/2009]

7. Global Forum for Health Research [www.globalforumhealth.org Accessed 21/7/2009]
8. International Union for Scientific Studies of Populations. [www.iussp.org Accessed 21/7/2009]
9. Feachem RGA. Poverty and inequity: a proper focus for the new century. Bull World Health Organ 2000; 78:1-2
10. Castro-Leal F, Dayton J, Demery L, Mehra K. Public spending on health in Africa: do the poor benefit? Bull World Health Organ 2000; 78:66-74
11. Gwatkin DR. health inequalities and the health of the poor: what we know? What can we do? Bull World Health Organ 2000; 3-18
12. Wagstaff A. socioeconomic inequalities in child mortality: comparisons across nine developing countries. Bull World Health Organ 2000; 78:19-29.
13. Gakidou EE, Murray CJL, Frenk J. Defining and measuring health inequality: an approach based on the distribution of health expectancy. Bull World Health Organ 2000; 78:42-54
14. Braveman P, Krieger N, Lynch J. Health inequalities and social inequalities in health. Bull World Health Organ 2000; 78:232-233
15. Wagstaff A. Poverty and health sector inequalities. Bull World Health Organ 2002; 80:97-105
16. Shibuya K, Boerma JT. LMeasuring progress towards reducing health inequalities. Bull World Health Organ 2005; 83:162-163
17. Braveman P, Starfield B, Geiger H Jack. World Health Report 2000: how it removes equity from the agenda for public health monitoring and policy. BMJ 2001; 323(7314): 678-681
18. Asada Y, Hedemann T. A Problem with the Individual Approach in the WHO Health Inequality Measurement. Int J Equity Health 2002 doi:10.1186/1475-9276-1-2 [http://www.equityhealthj.com/content/1/1/2]
19. Gwatkin DR, Rutstein S, Johnson K, Suliman E, Wagstaff A, Amouzou A. Socio-Economic Differences in Health, Nutrition, and Population within Developing Countries: An Overview. The World Bank 2007 HNP
20. Macinko A J, Starfield B. Annotated Bibliography on Equity in Health, 1980-2001. Measuring total health inequality: adding individual variation to group-level differences. Int J Equity Health 2002 doi:10.1186/1475-9276-1-1[ttp://www.equityhealthj.com/content/1/1/1]
21. Wagstaff A, Paci P, van Doorslaer E. On the measurement of inequalities in health. Soc Sci Med 1991; 33:545-557
22. Pamuk ER. Social class inequality in mortality from 1921 to 1972 in England a,nd Wales. Population Studies 1985; 39:17-31
23. Pamuk ER. Social class inequality in infant mortality in England and Wales from 1921 to 1980. Europ J Population 1988; 4:1-21
24. Kunst AE, Mackenbach JP. Measuring socio-economic inequalities in health. Copenhagen World Health Organization 1995
25. Mackenbach JP, Kunst AE. Measuring the magnitude of socio-economic inequalities in health: an overview of available measures illustrated with two examples from Europe. Soc Sci Med 1997; 44:757-771
26. Kunst AE, Mackenbach JP. International variation in the size of mortality differences associated with occupational status. Int J Epidemiol 1994; 23: 742-750
27. Kunst AE, Mackenbach JP. The size of mortality differences associated with educational level in nine industrialised countries. Am J Public Health 1994; 84:932-937.
28. Hayes LJ, Berry G. Sampling variability of the Kunst-Mackenbach relative index of inequality. J Epidemiol Community Health 2002; 56:762-765.
29. Murray CJL, Gakidou EE, Frenk J. Health inequalities and social group differences: what should we measure?: an approach based on the distribution of health expectancy. Bull World Health Organ 1999; 77:537-543
30. Gakidou EE, Murray CJL, Frenk J. Defining and measuring health inequality: an approach based on the distribution of health expectancy. Bull World Health Organ 2000; 78:42-54
31. Boutayeb A. The double burden of communicable and non communicable diseases in developing countries. Trans Roy Soc Trop Medicine Hygiene 2006; 100:191-199.
32. Starfield B. Improving equity in health: A research agenda. Int J Health Services 2001, 31(3):545-566
33. Williams RFG, Doessel DP. Measuring inequality: tools and an illustration. Int J Equity Health 2006 doi:10.1186/1475-9276-5-5 [http://www.equityhealthj.com/content/5/1/5]
34. Tugwell P, O'Connor A, Andersson N, Mhatre S, Kristjansson E, Jacobsen MJ et al. Reduction of inequalities in health: assessing evidence-based tools. Int J Equity Health 2006 doi:10-1186/1475-9276-5-11 [http://www.equityhealthj.com/content/5/1/11]
35. De Vogli R, Mistry R, Gnesotto R, Cornia GA. Has the relation between income inequality and life expectancy disappeared? Evidence from Italy and top industrialised countries. J Epidemiol Community Health 2005; 59: 158-162.
36. Gakidou E, King G. Measuring total health inequality: adding individual variation to group-level differences. Int J Equity Health 2002 doi:10.1186/1475-9276-1-3 [http://www.equityhealthj.com/content/1/1/3]
37. Scott V, Stern R, Sanders D, Reagon G, Mathews V. Research action to address inequalities: the experience of Cape Town Equity Gauge. Into J Equity Health 2008 doi:10.1186/1475-9276-7-6 [http://www.equityhealthj.com/content/7/1/6]
38. Signal L, Martin J, Reid P, Carroll C, Howden-Chapman, Ormsby VK et al. Tackling health inequalities: moving theory to action. Int J Equity Health 2007 doi:10.1186/1475-9276-6-12 [http://www.equityhealthj.com/content/6/1/12]
39. Mackenbach JP, Stirbu I, Roskam AJR, Schaap MM, Menvielle G, Leinsalu M et al, for the European Union Working Group on Socioeconomic Inequalities in Health. Socioeconomic Inequalities in Health in 22 European Countries. N Engl J Med 2008; 358:2468-81
40. Schuftan C. Poverty and Inequity in the Era of Globalization: Our Need to Change and to Re-conceptualize Int J Equity Health 2008 doi:1186/1475-9276-2-4 [http://www.equityhealthj.com/content/2/1/4]
41. Heggenhougen HK. The epidemiology of inequity: Will research make a difference? Norsk Epidemiologi 2005; 15:127-132
42. Reidpath DD, Allotey P. Measuring global health inequity. Int J Equity Health 2007 doi:10.1186/1475-9276-6-16 [http://www.equityhealthj.com/content/6/1/16]
43. Gwatckin DR. The need for equity-oriented health sector reforms. Into J epidemiology 2001; 30:720-723
44. Low A, Ithindi T, Low A. A step too far? Making health equity interventions in Namibia more sufficient. Int J Equity Health 2003 doi:10.1186/1475-9276-2-5 [http://www.equityhealthj.com/content/2/1/5]
45. Van de Poel E, Hosseinpoor AR, Jehu-Appiah C, Vega J, Speybroeck N. Malnutrition and the disproportional burden on the poor: the case of Ghana. Int J Equity Health 2007 doi:10.1186/1475-9276-6-21 [http://www.equityhealthj.com/content/6/1/21]
46. Zere E, Mandlhate C, Mbeeli T, Shangula K, Mutirua K, Kapenambili W. Equity in health care in Namibia: developing a needs-based resource allocation formula using principal components analysis. Int J Equity Health 2007, 6:3 doi:10.1186/1475-9276-6-3 [http://www.equityhealthj.com/content/6/1/3]
47. Yiengprugsawan V, Lim LLY, Carmichael GA, Sidorenko A, Sleigh AC. Measuring and decomposing inequity in self-reported morbidity and self-assessed health in Thailand. Int J Equity Health 2007 doi:10.1186/1475-9276-6-23 [http://www.equityhealthj.com/content/6/1/23]
48. Mackenbach JP, Stronks K. The development of a strategy for tackling health inequalities in the Netherlands. Int J Equity Health 2003 doi:10.1186/1475-9276-3-11 [http://www.equityhealthj.com/content/3/1/11]
49. Garenne M, Hohmann-Garenne S. A Wealth Index to Screen High-risk Families: Application to Morocco. J Health Popul Nutr 2003; 21: 235-242
50. Marmot M, on behalf of the Commission on Social Determinants of Health. Achieving health equity: from root causes to fair outcomes. Lancet 2007; 370:1153-1163
51. Marmot M, Friel S. Global health equity: evidence for action on the social determinants of health. J Epidemiol Community Health 2008;62:1095-1097
52. Watts S, Siddiqi S. Social Determinants of Health in the Eastern Mediterranean Region: A discussion paper. Division of Health Systems and Services Development WHO, EMRO 2006
53. Schofield T. Health inequity and its social determinants: A sociological commentary. Health Sociology Review 2007; 16(2):105-114
54. Tugwell P, Petticrew M, Robinson V, Kristjansson E, Maxwell L, for the Cochrane Equity Field Editorial Team. Cochrane and Campbell Collaborations, and health equity. Lancet 2006; 367:1128-1130

55. Kunst AE, Bos V, Lahelma E, Bartley M, Lissau I, Regidor E et al. Trends in socioeconomic inequalities in self-assessed health in 10 European countries. Intern J Epidemiology 2005; 34(2):295-305
56. van Lenthe FJ, Borrell LN, Costa G, Roux AVD, Kauppinen TM, Marinacci C et al. Neighbourhood unemployment and all cause mortalmity: a comparison of six countries. J Epiemiol Community Health 2005; 56: 231-237.
57. Merlo J, Gerdtham ULF-G, Lynch J, Beckman A, Norlund A, Lithman T. Social inequalities in health- do they diminish with age? Revisiting the question in Sweden 1999. Int J Equity Health 2004 doi:10.1186/1475-9276-2-2 [http://www.equityhealthj.com/content 2/1/2]
58. Boutayeb A. Social inequality and health inequity in Morocco. Int J Equity Health 2006 doi:10.1186/1475-9276-5-1 [http://www.equityhealthj.com/content 5/1/1]
59. Valle AM. Social class, marginality and self-assessed health: a cross-sectional analysis of the health gradient in Mexico. Int J Equity Health 2009 doi:10.1186/1475-9276-8-3 [http://www.equityhealthj.com/content/8/1/3]
60. Sun X, Rehnberg C, Meng O. How are individual-level social capital and poverty associated with health equity. A study from Chinese cities. doi:10.1186/1475-9276-8-2 [http://www.equityhealthj.com/content/8/1/2]
61. Shawky S. Infant mortality in Arab countries: sociodemographic, perinatal and economic factors. East Mediter Health J 2001; 7(6): 956-965
62. Amone J, Asio S, Cattaneo A, Kweyatulira AK, Macaluso A , Maciocco G et al , Maurice Mukokoma, Luca Ronfani, Stefano Santini. User fees in private non-for-profit hospitals in Uganda: a survey and intervention for equity. Int J Eq Health 2005. doi:10.1186/1475-9276-6-21[http://www.equityhealthj.com/content/6/1/21]
63. Solomon NM. Health information generation and utilization for informed decision-making in equitable health service management: The case of Kenya Partnership for Health program. Int J Equity Health 2005 doi:10.1186/1475-9276-4-8 [http://www.equityhealthj.com/content/4:1/8].
64. Singh S, Dahal K, Mills E. Nepal's War on Human Rights: A summit higher than Everest. Int J Equity Health 2005 doi:10.1186/1475-9276-4-9 [http://www.equityhealthj.com/content/4/1/9]
65. Boutayeb A, Boutayeb S The burden of non communicable diseases in developing countries. Int J Equity Health 2005 doi:10.1186/1475-9276-4-2 [http://www.equityhealthj.com/content/4/1/2]
66. Boutayeb A. Developing countries and neglected diseases: challenges and perspectives. Int J Equity Health 2007 doi:10.1186/1475-9276-6-20 [http://www.equityhealthj.com/content/6/1/20]
67. Essien EJ, Ross MW, Williams ML, Meshack AF, Fernández-Esquer ME, Peters RJ, Ogungbade GO. Primary source of income is associated with differences in HIV risk behaviors in street-recruited samples. Int J Equity Health 2004 doi:10.1186/1475-9276-3-5 [http://www.equityhealthj.com/content/3/1/5]
68. Gupta N, Zurn P, Diallo K, Poz MRD.Primary source of income is associated with differences in HIV risk behaviours in street-recruited samples. Int J Equity Health 2003 doi:10.1186/1475-9276-2-11 [http://www.equityhealthj.com/content/2/1/11]]
69. Uzochukwu BSC, Onwujekwe OE.Socio-economic differences and health seeking behaviour for the diagnosis and treatment of malaria: a case study of four local government areas operating the Bamako initiative programme in south-east Nigeria. Int J Equity Health 2004 doi:10.1186/1475-9276-3-6 [http://www.equityhealthj.com/content/3/1/6]
70. Mathanga DP, Bowie C. Malaria control in Malawi: are the poor being served? Int J Equity Health 2007 doi:10.1186/1475-9276-6-22 [http://www.equityhealthj.com/content/6/1/22]
71. Simwaka BN, Bello G, Banda H, Chimzizi R, Squire BSB, Theobald SJ. The Malawi National Tuberculosis Programme: an equity analysis. Int J Equity Health doi:10.1186/1475-9276-6-24 [http://www.equityhealthj.com/content/6/1/24
72. Antunes JLF, Pérez CBC, Boing AF, Wünsch-Filho V. Inequalities in mortality of men by oral and pharyngeal cancer in Barcelona, Spain and São Paulo, Brazil, 1995–2003. Int J Equity Health 2008. doi:10.1186/1475-9276-7-14 http://www.equityhealthj.com/content/7/1/14]
73. Klassen AC, Smith KC, Shariff-Marco S, Juon HS.A healthy mistrust: how worldview relates to attitudes about breast cancer screening in a cross-sectional survey of low-income women. Int J Equity Health 2008 doi:10.1186/1475-9276-7-15 http://www.equityhealthj.com/content/7/1/5]
74. Goyder E, Dibben C, Grimsley M, Peters J, Blank L, Ellis E. Variation in prescribing for anxiety and depression: a reflection of health inequalities, cultural differences or variations in access to care? Int J Equity Health 2006 doi:10.1186/1475-9276-6-21 [http://www.equityhealthj.com/content/6/1/21]
75. Boutayeb A. Health and Soustainable Development. University Mohamed Ier Press, 2004.
76. Houweling TAJ, Kunst AE, Mackenbach JP. Measuring health inequality among children in developing countries: does the choice of the indicator of economic status matter? Intern J Eq Health 2003 doi:10.1186/1475-9276-2-8 [http://www.equityhealthj.com/content/2/1/8]
77. Van de Poel E Hosseinpoor AR Speybroeck N Ourti TV Vega J. Socioeconomic inequality in malnutrition in developing countries. Bull of the World Health Organization 2007; 86(14): 282-291
78. Houweling TAJ, Kunst AE, Huisman M, Mackenbach JP. Using relative and absolute measures for monitoring health inequalities: experiences from cross-national analyses on maternal and child health. Int J Equity Health 2007 doi:10.1186/1475-9276-6-15 [http://www.equityhealthj.com/content/6/1/15]
79. Fotso JC. Child health inequities in developing countries: differences across urban and rural areas. Int J Equity Health 2006 doi:10.1186/1475-9276-6-17 [http://www.equityhealthj.com/content/6/1/17]
80. Khawaja M, Dawns J, Meyerson-Knox S, Yamout.R. Disparities in child health in the Arab region during the 1990s. Int J Equity Health 2008 doi:10.1186/1475-9276-7-14 [http://www.equityhealthj.com/content/7/1/14]
81. Chen E, Martin AD, Matthews KA. Socioeconomic status and health: Do gradients differ within childhood and adolescence. Soc Sci Med 2006; 62-2161-2170
82. Case A, Fertig A Paxson C. The lasting impact of childhood health and circumstance. J Health Economics 2005; 24:365-389
83. Zere E, McIntyre D. Inequities in under-five child malnutrition in South Africa. Int J Equity Health 2003 doi:10.1186/1475-9276-2-7 [http://www.equityhealthj.com/content/2/1/7]
84. Wamani H, Tylleskär T, Åstrøm AN, Tumwine JK, Peterson S. Mothers' education but not fathers' education, household assets or land ownership is the best predictor of child health inequalities in rural Uganda. Int J Equity Health 2004 doi:10.1186/1475-9276-3-9 [http://www.equityhealthj.com/content/3/1/9]
85. Hong R, Banta JE, Betancourt JA. Relationship between household wealth inequality and chronic childhood under-nutrition in Bangladesh. Int J Equity Health 2006 doi:10.1186/1475-9276-5-15 [http://www.equityhealthj.com/content/5/1/15]
86. Razzaque A, Streatfield PK, Gwatkin DR. Does health intervention improve socioeconomic inequalities of neonatal, infant and child mortality? Evidence from Matlab Bangladesh. Int J Equity Health 2007 doi:10.1186/1475-9276-6-4 [http://www.equityhealthj.com/content/6/1/4]
87. Giashuddin SM, Rahman A, Rahman F, Mashrekey SR, Chowdhury SM, Linnan M, Safinaz S. Socioeconomic inequality in child injury in Bangladesh - implication for developing countries. Int J Equity Health 2009 doi:10.1186/1475-9276-8-7 [http://www.equityhealthj.com/content/8/1/7]
88. Khun S, Manderson L. Zhu JM, Zhu Y, Liu R. Health insurance of rural/township schoolchildren in Pinggu, Beijing: coverage rate, determinants, disparities, and sustainability. Int J Equity Health 2008 doi:10.1186/1475-9276-7-23 [http://www.equityhealthj.com/content/7/1/23]
89. Zhu JM, Zhu Y, Liu R. Health insurance of rural/township schoolchildren in Pinggu, Beijing: coverage rate, determinants, disparities, and sustainability. Int J Equity Health 2008 doi:10.1186/1475-9276-7-23 [http://www.equityhealthj.com/content/7/1/23]
90. Boutayeb A. Maternal mortality in Morocco 2009[www.iussp.org/2009 conference]

91. Say L, Raine R. A systematic review of inequalities in the use of maternal health care in developing countries: examining the scale of the problem and the importance of context. Bull World Health Organ 2007; 85(10):812-819

92. Islam M. The Safe Motherhood Initiative and beyond. Bull World Health Organ 2007; 85(10):735-735

93. Houweling TAJ, Ronsmans C, Campbell OMC, Kunst AE. Huge poor-rich inequalities in maternity care: an international comparative study of maternity and child care in developing countries. Bul World Health Org. Bull World Health Org 2007; 85:745-754

94. Collin SM, Anwar I, Ronsmans C. A decade of inequality in maternity care: antenatal care, professional attendance at delivery, and caesarean section in Bangladesh (1991–2004). Int J Equity Health 2007 doi:10.1186/1475-9276-6-9 [http://www.equityhealthj.com/content/6/1/9]

95. Lanre-Abass BA. Poverty and maternal mortality in Nigeria: towards a more viable ethics of modern medical practice. Int J Equity Health 2008 doi:10.1186/1475-9276-7-11 [http://www.equityhealthj.com/content/7/1/11]

96. Andersson N, Ho-Foster A .13,915 reasons for equity in sexual offences legislation: A national school-based survey in South Africa. Int J Equity Health 2008 doi:10.1186/1475-9276-7-20 [http://www.equityhealthj.com/content/7/1/20]

97. Joffres C, Mills E, Joffres M, Khanna T, Walia H, Grund D. Sexual slavery without borders: trafficking for commercial sexual exploitation in India. Int J Equity Health 2008 doi:10.1186/1475-9276-6-22 [http://www.equityhealthj.com/content/6/1/22]

98. Demirchyan A, Thompson ME. Demirchyan A, Thompson ME. .Determinants of self-rated health in women: a population-based study in Armavir Marz, Armenia, 2001 & 2004. Intern J Eq Health 2008 doi:10.1186/1475-9276-7-25 [http://www.equityhealthj.com/content/7/1/25]

99. Boutayeb A, Serghini M. Health Indicators and human development in the Arab Region. Int J Health Geogr doi:10-1186/1476-072X-5-61[http://www.ij-healthgeographics.com/content/5/1/61]

100. Gupta N, Zurn P, Diallo K, Dal Poz MR. Uses of population census data for monitoring geographical imbalance in the health workforce: snapshots from three developing countries. Int J Equity Health doi:10.1186/1475-9276-5-13 [http://www.equityhealthj.com/content/5/1/13]

101. Le Cai, Chongsuvivatwong V. Rural-urban differentials of premature mortality burden in south-west China. Int J Equity Health 2006 doi:10.1186/1475-9276-5-13 [http://www.equityhealthj.com/content/5/1/13]

102. Kazembe LN, Appleton CC, Kleinschmidt I. Geographical disparities in core population coverage indicators for roll back malaria in Malawi. Intern J Eq Health 2007 doi:10.1186/1475-9276-6-5 [http://www.equityhealthj.com/content/6/1/5]

103. Perry HB, King-Schultz LW, Aftab AS, Bryant JH. Health equity issues at the local level: Socio-geography, access, and health outcomes in the service area of the Hôpital Albert Schweitzer-Haiti. Int J Equity Health 2007 doi:10.1186/1475-9276-6-7 [http://www.equityhealthj.com/content/6/1/7]

104. Ben Romdhane H, Grenier F R. Social determinants in Tunisia: the case-analysis of Ariana. Int J Equity Health 2009 doi:1186/1475-9276-8-9 [http://www.equityhealthj.com/content/8/1/9]

105. Sadler GR, Ryujin L, Nguyen T, Oh G, Paik G, Kustin B. Heterogeneity within the Asian American community. Int J Equity Health 2008 doi:10.1186/1475-9276-2-12 [http://www.equityhealthj.com/content/2/1/12]

106. Ronellenfitsch U, Razum O Deteriorating health satisfaction among immigrants from Eastern Europe to Germany. Int J Equity Health 2003 doi:10.1186/1475-9276-3-4 [http://www.equityhealthj.com/content/3/1/4]

107. Syed HR, Dalgard OS, Hussain A, Dalen I, Claussen B, Ahlberg NL. Inequalities in health: a comparative study between ethnic Norwegians and Pakistanis in Oslo, Norway. Int J Equity Health 2006 doi:10.1186/1475-9276-5-7 [http://www.equityhealthj.com/content/5/1/7]

108. Bekker MHJ, Lhajoui M. Health and literacy in first- and second-generation Moroccan Berber women in the Netherlands: Ill literacy? Int J Equity Health 2004 doi:10.1186/1475-9276-3-8 [http://www.equityhealthj.com/content/3/1/8]

109. Kelaher M, Paul S, Lambert H, Ahmad W, Smith GD. The applicability of measures of socioeconomic position to different ethnic groups within the UK. Int J Equity Health [http://www.equityhealthj.com/content/8/1/4]

110. Yu CP, Whynes DK, Sach TH. Equity in health care financing: The case of Malaysia. Int J Equity Health 2005 doi:10.1186/1475-9276-7-15 [http://www.equityhealthj.com/content/7/1/15]

111. Levy JI, Chemerynski SM, Tuchmann JL. Incorporating concepts of inequality and inequity into health benefits analysis. Int J Equity Health 2006 doi:10.1186/1475-9276-5-2 [http://www.equityhealthj.com/content/5/1/2]

CHAPTER 4

Equity and Disease Burden

Abdesslam Boutayeb

*Department of Mathematics Faculty of Sciences, Boulevard Mohamed VI, BP: 717 Oujda, Morocco,
Email: x.boutayeb@menara.ma*

Abstract: The contrast between life expectancy of 43 years for a woman in sub-Saharan Africa compared with 86 years for a woman in Japan is inconceivable and unfair. This is not a mere inequality it is one kind of health inequities existing between developed and developing countries. A multitude of other such health inequities are given by maternal mortality, infant mortality, diseases burden and access to different basic health services such as vaccination, antenatal care, postnatal visits, hospital beds, number of health personnel. Health inequity, however, is not a special feature characterizing the difference between rich and poor countries, neither is poor health confined to those worst off. In all countries, independently of their income and level of development, health and illness follow a social gradient. For instance, in the U.K, the 28 year life expectancy gap between men living in two different cities is incredible.

Keywords: Health (in)equity, maternal mortality, child mortality, life expectancy, developed countries, developing countries

1. INTRODUCTION

During the last century, several declarations and conventions were adopted on the rights of children, men and women to have a decent healthy life, free of hunger, violence and ignorance [see chapter on health and child rights in this book]. In particular, the Universal Declaration of Human Rights (1948) proclaimed that "All human beings are born free and equal in dignity and rights. They are endowed with reason and conscience and should act towards one another in a sprit of brotherhood" [1], whereas the first article of Geneva Declaration of the Rights of the Child stipulates that "The child that is hungry must be fed; the child that is sick must be nursed; the child that is backward must be helped; the delinquent child must be reclaimed; and the orphan and the waif must be sheltered and succoured" [2]. Unfortunately, despite the efforts devoted by international organisms such as the World Health Organization, the UNICEF, UNESCO and others, the third millennium is witnessing growing and unacceptable inequalities in health outputs and access to health services. The distribution of disease burden expressed in terms of mortality and morbidity is uneven. The gap between developed and developing countries is questioning the humanity. It has become an ethical issue. However, this is only one side of the problem. The other challenge is facing governments and decision makers within each country of the globe.

2. HEALTH INEQUITY: A GLOBAL MULTIDIMENSIONAL PROBLEM

Worldwide, between and within countries, health inequities follow a socioeconomic gradient. As expressed by the WHO Director-General in the overview of the WHO Report 2003, inequalities between rich and poor span the whole life cycle. They affect life expectancy, the healthy life, nutrition, access to basic health services such as vaccination, hospital beds, antenatal care, postnatal visits, as well as access to other basic needs like education, drinking water and improved sanitation [3](see box).

[Box WHO Director-General in the overview, WHO report 2003]

While a baby girl born in Japan today can expect to live for about 85 years, a girl born at the same moment in Sierra Leone has a life expectancy of 36 years. The Japanese child will receive vaccinations, adequate nutrition and good schooling. If she becomes a mother she will benefit from high-quality maternity care. Growing older, she may eventually develop chronic diseases, but excellent treatment and rehabilitation services will be available; she can expect to receive, on average, medications worth about US$ 550 per year and much more if needed.

Meanwhile, the girl in Sierra Leone has little chance of receiving immunizations and high probability of being underweight throughout childhood. She will probably marry in adolescence and go on to give birth to six or more children without assistance of a trained birth attendant. One or more of her babies will die in infancy, and she herself will be at high risk of death in childbirth. If she falls ill, she can expect, on average, medicines worth about US$3 per year. If she survives middle age she, too, will develop chronic diseases but, without access to adequate treatment, she will die prematurely.

[End Box]

3. HEALTH INEQUITY BETWEEN COUNTRIES

3.1 Life expectancy and healthy life expectancy

In High income countries, life expectancy at birth was estimated at 80 years in 2005 [4], compared to less than 60 years in low income countries, yielding a 30 years global gap. Moreover, another dimension of inequity is added when comparing the quality of life. Indeed, the ratio of healthy life expectancy to life expectancy is greater in rich countries (0.89) than in poor countries (0.85) (Table **1**)

Table 1. Health expectancy and healthy life expectancy by income group of countries

Income group Indicator	Low income	Lower middle income	Upper middle income	High income
Life expectancy Birth (LEB) (years)	59	71	69	80
Healthy life expectancy at birth (HALE) (years)	50	62	63	71
Ratio HALE/LEB	0.85	0.87	0.91	0.89

3.2 Maternal mortality and infant mortality

The fourth and fifth Millennium Development Goals (MDGs) aim to reduce mortality in children under age five by two third and maternal mortality by three quarter between 1990 and 2015 [5].

Monitoring the coverage of priority interventions to achieve these two goals, the Countdown to 2015 for Maternal, Newborn, and child Survival initiative was launched in order to monitor achievements of the two goals. The first round of the Countdown reported in 2005 on 60 countries and 17 interventions, focusing on child survival. According to the 2008 report released on "tracking coverage of interventions"[6], 68 countries have 97% of maternal and child death worldwide. The World Health Statistics 2008 [4] show that neonatal, infant and children under five mortality rates in low income countries are respectively 10, 12 and 16 times higher than in high income countries (Table **2**). The inequalities are more pronounced if a country like Liberia which have rates at 66, 157 and 235, is compared to Japan with rates 1, 3 and 4.

Table 2. Maternal, neonatal, infant and children mortality by income group of countries

Income group Indicator	Low income	Lower middle income	Upper middle income	High income
MMR (per 1 00 000 live births)	650	180	91	9
Neonatal Mortality rate (per 1000 live births)	40	19	12	4
IMR (per 1000 live births)	73	27	22	6
U5MR (per 1000 live births)	110	35	26	7

As expressed by the report released by the House of Commons International Development Committee in UK in 2008, of all health measures, maternal mortality indicators represent the greatest gap between rich and poor countries [7]. The report indicates that one in seven women in Niger can expect to die in childbirth, compared to one in 8200 in the UK. This is more than a 1000 fold difference. The estimates for maternal mortality in 2005, developed jointly by WHO, UNICEF, UNFPA and the World Bank are appalling [8]. Not surprisingly, Maternal Mortality Ratio (MMR) was found to be higher in developing regions (at 450 maternal deaths per 100 000 live births), in stark contrast to developed regions (at 9 maternal deaths per 100 000 live births). Among the developing regions, sub-Sahara Africa had the highest MMR (at 900 maternal deaths per 100 000 live births), followed by South Asia(490), Oceania (430), South-Eastern Asia (300), Western Asia (160), Northern Africa (160), Latin America and the Caribbean (130), and Eastern Asia (50). The gap appears more profound when comparing a country like Sierra Leone having a MMR of 2100 to a country like Ireland which had a MMR of 1.

More globally, the World Health Statistics show that in 2006 Low income countries had a MMR of 650 compared to 9 in high income countries (Table **2**).

3.3 Inequity in mortality caused by specific diseases

With malnutrition as a common contributor, the five biggest infectious killers in the world are acute respiratory infections, HIV/AIDS, diarrhoea, malaria and tuberculosis, responsible for nearly 80% of the total infectious disease burden and claiming about 12 million people per year. As indicated in Table 3, developing countries bear the quasi totality of these diseases toll [9].

Table 3. Main causes of Mortality due to infectious diseases, 2001(in million)

Disease	Deaths per year	% Developing countries
Respiratory infections	3.9	80%
AIDS	3.	90%
Diarrhoeal diseases	1.9	90%
Tuberculosis	1.9	50%
Malaria	1.1	90%

Moreover, poor countries are not only specially affected by communicable diseases which are often related to poverty but also compete with rich countries on injuries and non communicable diseases like cardiovascular diseases, diabetes and cancer, once known as diseases of the rich. According to the World Health Statistics 2008 [4], it appears that mortality caused by AIDS and tuberculosis is about 20 times higher in low income countries than in high income countries. The mortalities caused by non communicable diseases and injuries in poor regions are nearly twice and three times higher than in rich regions (Table **4**).

Table 4. Mortality rates for specific diseases by income group of countries

Income group Mortality Rate	Low income	Lower middle Income	Upper middle income	High income
HIV/AIDS (per 100 000)	58	10	70	3
Tuberculosis (per 100 000)	43	18	21	2
NCD (per 100 000)	754	668	728	419
CVD (per 100 000)	418	324	436	173
Cancer (per 100 000)	114	136	138	136
Injuries (per 100 000)	116	81	102	42

3.4 Disease Burden and Health Equity

Beyond mortality statistics, different methods can be considered to quantify the burden of disease expressed in terms of socio-economic costs such as productivity losses, care and treatment, hospitalization and handicap. In order to overcome the specific problems of each country, the most used method is the approach that measures the global burden of disease in terms of Disability Adjusted Life Years (DALYs) which is a combination of Years of Life Lost (YLL) through premature death, and Years Lived with Disability (YLD). Thus, DALY is thought of as one lost year of healthy life [10]. Table 5 shows the distribution of disease burden by age and regions. The gap between developed and developing countries is specially illustrated in child mortality. In high-mortality developing countries, 49% of the disease burden is caused by deaths under age 15, compared to 10% in developed countries.

Table 5. Distribution of disease burden (DALYs) by age group and region, 2002

Age group Region	0-4 (%)	5-14 (%)	15-59 (%)	60+ (%)
Developed	6	4	57	33
Low-mortality developing	18	6	57	19
High-mortality developing	40	9	43	8
World	29	7	49	15

In a critical analysis of the way of measuring global heath inequity, Reidpath and Allotey considered the disease burden in 2000, indicating that, worldwide, there were 0.247 DALYs per capita [11]. Regionally, however, the distribution was uneven varying from 0.129 DALYs per capita in EUROA to 0.635 DALYs per capita in AFROE. Under the assumption of equality of disease burden, the ratio between poor and rich region is about 5. Instead of assuming that it would be equitable for each region to achieve identical DALYs per capita (i.e., .247 per capita), the authors assumed that each region should achieve a level of DALYs per capita in proportion to its capita wealth. WPROA has a per capita wealth of $23,685 whereas AFROE has a per capita wealth $1802. Under this form of equity the wealthiest region would be expected to experience a per capita DALYs level of 13.14 times that of the poorest region.

4. HEALTH INEQUITY WITHIN COUNTRIES

Worldwide, from the slums of India and remote villages of Brazil and Iran to capitals of Norway, Canada, England and Australia, governments and decision makers are challenged by inadmissible health inequities arising as unfair and unjust inequalities due mainly to social determinants which can be tackled. The report published jointly in 2008 by the World Health Organization and the Public Health Agency of Canada gives examples of inter-sectoral action on health and health equity in 18 countries [12].

4.1 Life expectancy: mind the step!

Beyond the gaps between developed and developing countries, unfair inequalities are found within all countries, independently of their level of development. As expressed by Marmot and Friel [13], two figures captured attention by the report of the Commission on Social Determinants of Health published in 2008 [14, see box]. The first was the contrast between life expectancy of 43 for a woman in Zambia compared with 86 for a woman in Japan. The second was the 28 year life expectancy gap between men in Calton in Glasgow and men in Lenzie 13 km away. If the gap of 43 years in life expectancy between a woman in a developed region and another in a developing country is inconceivable, the 28 years difference in life expectancy in a same country like UK is incredible.

[Box Commission on Social Determinants of Health [14]]

"Our children have dramatically different life chances depending on where they were born. In Japan or Sweden they can expect to live more than 80 years; in Brazil, 72 years; India, 63 years; and in one of several African countries, fewer than 50 years. And within countries, the differences in life chances are dramatic and seen worldwide. The poorest of the poor have high levels of illness and premature mortality. But poor health is not confined to those worst off. In countries at all levels of income, health and illness follow a social gradient: the lower the socioeconomic position, the worse the health.

[End Box]

4.2 Maternal mortality and infant mortality

There is no doubt that children from the poorest 20% of population are more likely to die before their fifth birthday than those living in the wealthiest 20% households. A similar statement can be made for women dying during pregnancy and labour. During the last decade or so, an abundant literature was especially devoted to the study of health inequities associated with children mortality and the social determinants underlying it.

According to the State of the World's Children 2006 "Excluded and Invisible", over 5.5 million children under five die every year from causes related to malnutrition, whereas vaccine–preventable diseases cause more than 2 million deaths every year, of which approximately 1.4 million occur in children under age five [15]. The report stresses that in 13 countries where data are available, children from the poorest 20 per cent of the population are more than twice as likely to be underweight for their age. In Lesotho and Swaziland they are respectively three and five times as likely to be underweight. A similar pattern of inequity was seen in immunization coverage showing that, in Chad, Azerbaijan, Democratic Republic of Congo and Sudan (North), rich children were twice as likely to be vaccinated against measles compared to poor children. In Niger and Central African Republic, the ratio was 3 and nearly 4 respectively. Consequently and obviously, poor children are more likely to die during their childhood than rich children. The ratio is between 2 and 3 in several countries, reaching 4 in South Africa and exceeding 5 in Peru.

Houweling *et al* considered Demographic and Health Surveys data from ten countries (Bolivia, Brazil, Indonesia, Cameroon, Chad, Kenya, Malawi, Pakistan, Tanzania and Uganda), comparing between 4 different indicators to measure poor-rich inequalities in under five mortality and measles immunization coverage [16]. They concluded that researchers should be very careful when comparing results of studies using different indices. However, despite the sensitivity of the magnitude of inequality to the use of different indices, all countries considered showed a significant level of inequity in mortality between children from the poorest quintile and those belonging to the richest quintile. For instance children mortality rates in Bolivia were in the range 126.2-135.1 for the poorest quintile whereas they were in the range 28.8-32.7 the in richest quintile. In Malawi they ranged between 193.4 and 259.2 in the poorest quintile compared to a range 157.3-176.1 in the richest quintile.

Using component analysis and a generalization of the concentration index to analyse data from 47 developing countries, Vand de Poel *et al* have shown that socioeconomic inequality in malnutrition is present throughout these countries [17]. Estimating stunting and wasting rates in children aged less than five years according to socioeconomic status the authors illustrated clearly the differences between children belonging to the wealthiest quintiles compared to those from the poorest quintiles. As shown in Table 6, children from poorest socioeconomic households are more likely to be stunted than those from the richest families. In countries like Cameroon, Ghana, Nigeria, Bangladesh, Pakistan and Morocco, poor children are about twice times exposed to stunting compared to children from the wealthiest quintile. The ratio reaches 3.4, 3.8 and 4.5 in Bolivia, Peru and Nicaragua respectively, skyrocketing at 6.8 in Turkey.

Table 6. Prevalence of stunting rates in selected countries (for children under five years of age)

Quintile Country	Q1 (Poorest) (%)	Q1 (middle) (%)	Q1 (richest) (%)	Ratio Q1 / Q3
Cameroon	44.19	38.85	19.20	2.3
Ghana	45.11	40.42	20.01	2.2
Nigeria	54.30	49.55	25.20	2.2
Bangladesh	58.19	53.32	30.26	1.9
Pakistan	61.91	53.58	35.98	1.7
Morocco	34.87	20.07	16.02	2.2
Turkey	34.25	17.48	5.01	6.8
Bolivia	48.50	29.68	14.29	3.4
Nicaragua	42.16	22.14	9.46	4.5
Peru	54.91	24.91	14.36	3.8

Data from Egypt, Morocco and Tunisia indicate that for immunization coverage, inequalities are generally attenuated between rural and urban areas, rich and poor families, as well as between developed and deprived regions [18-20]. This achievement is mainly due to national and international efforts based on generalised policies of public health with specified targets aiming to reach deprived and vulnerable populations. At the opposite side, health outputs like infant and child mortality, stunting and underweight all show unjustifiable gaps between rural and urban; poor and rich; developed and deprived regions; and illiterate and educated women. Exacerbated inequalities are found in health outputs, the pattern of inequalities in Egypt and Morocco are similar. The poorest children (respectively infant) are three time (respectively two and half) likely to die than the richest children and infant. Stunting and under weight reveal similar levels of inequality, with a fourfold gap in Moroccan underweight (17/4) (Figures **1** and **2**).

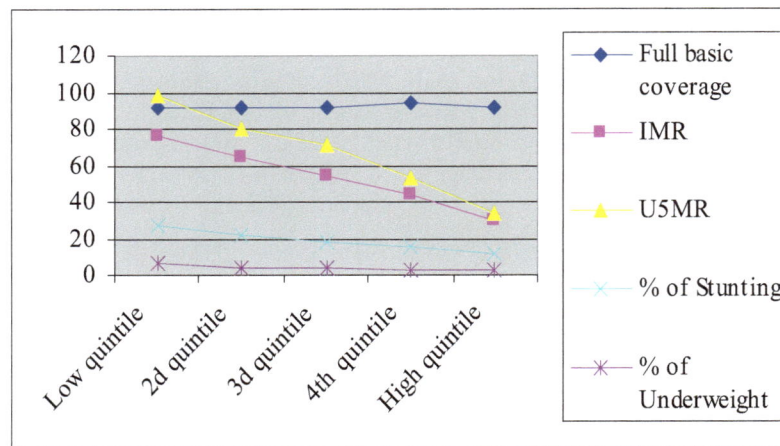

Figure 1. Health indicators in Egypt.

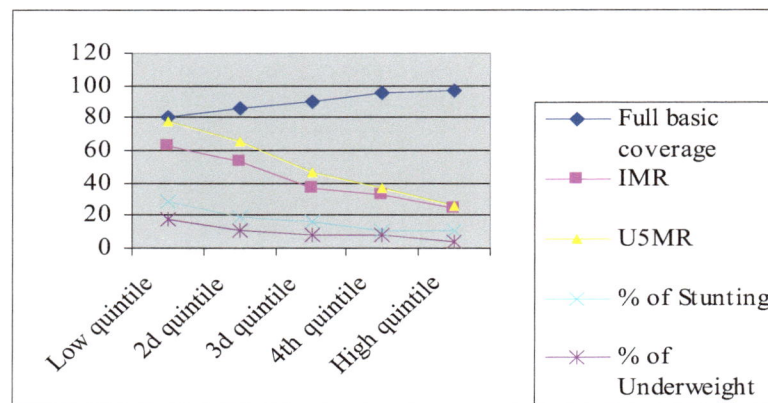

Figure 2. Health indicators in Morocco.

In Libya, effect of socioeconomic factors on child development were considered in a cross-sectional study carried out in two regions (Al Jabel and Tripoli) of the Jamahiriya on the growth and nutritional status of children under 5 years of age. The prevalence of stunting was higher among Al Jabel children (6·1%) than in Tripoli (2·5%) and in rural (6·8%) rather than urban (2·8%) areas [21].

Using available data from national household surveys of 18 Arab countries, Khawaja *et al* analysed the impact of socioeconomic factors on child mortality and morbidity. Child health was measured by nutritional status, vaccination and Acute Respiratory Infection. Gender, residence (urban/rural), maternal education level, per capita GDP, female literacy rates, urban population and doctors per 100 000 inhabitants were used to describe and analyse within-country disparities in child health. The authors concluded that disparity by place of residence showed significantly higher rates of child mortality in rural areas and a similar trend in nutritional status. Whereas absence of gender disparity was noticed in immunization coverage. A noticeable disadvantage of illiterate mothers compared to mothers with at least secondary education was seen in wasting, stunting and vaccination rates. Egypt, Morocco and Tunisia were among the countries with largest disparity [22].

Using the concentration index to analyse child mortality and morbidity caused by infectious diseases, non communicable diseases and injury among 1-4 years children in Bangladesh, Giashuddin *et al* found that children from poorest families were more likely to suffer from mortality and morbidity than richest children [23].

5. CONCLUSION

At the beginning of the third millennium, worldwide, unfair inequalities are worldwide persistent or even increasing. The gaps between developed and developing countries are inadmissible. But within countries, developing and developed alike, unjust differences are also incredible. The multidimensional spectre of inequity is illustrated by different health indicators such as maternal mortality ratio, infant mortality rate, proportion of population with access to health services, improving water and sanitation. Despite gains in average population health throughout the world, strategies based on average numbers like the Millennium Development Goals may improve health indicators globally without reducing inequities between rural and urban populations or between groups of different socioeconomic status. As stressed by the Commission on Social Determinants of Health, social justice is a matter of life or death.

6. CONFLICT INTERSET

The authors declare that they have no conflict interest

7. ACKNOWLEDGEMENTS

This paper was partly supported by a grant under the Global Project for Research (PGR) of the University Mohamed Premier, Oujda.

8. REFERENCES

1. United Nations. Universal Declaration of Human Rights. Geneva. 1948 [http://www.un.org/Overview/rights.html Accessed 1 April 2009]
2. Geneva Declaration on the Rights of the Child 1924 [http://www.un-documents.net/gdrc1924.htm Accessed 2 April 2009]
3. WHO. The World Health Report 2003: Shaping the Future. World Health Organization Geneva, 2003a.
4. WHO. The World Health Statistics 2008. World Health Organization Geneva, 2008.
5. UN. United Nations Millennium Declaration. New York, NY, United Nations, 2000
6. Countdown Coverage Writing Group. Countdown to 2015 for maternal, newborn, and child survival: the 2008 report on tracking coverage of interventions. Lancet 2008; 371: 1247-1258
7. House of Commons International Development Committee. Maternal Health: Fifth report of Session 2007-2008. London: The Stationery Office Limited 2007
8. WHO: Maternal Mortality: estimated by WHO, UNICEF, UNFPA, and the World Bank. Geneva: World Heal(9th Organization 2007
9. WHO. Global defence against the infectious diseases threat. Geneva: World Health Organization 2003b
10. Boutayeb A. The burden of communicable and non communicable diseases in developing countries. Trans. R Soc Trop Med Hyg 2006; 100: 191-199
11. Reidpath DD Allotey P. Measuring global health inequity. Int J Equity Health 2007; 6: 16
12. WHO. Health Equity Through Intersectoral Action: An Analysis of 18 Country Case Studies. Geneva: World Health Organization 2008
13. Marmot M Friel S. Global health equity: evidence for action on the social determinants of health. J Epidemiol Community Health 2008; 62:1095–97
14. Commission on Social Determinants of health. Closing the gap in a generation: health equity through action on the social determinants of health. Geneva: World Health Organization, 2008
15. UNICEF: The state of the world's children: Excluded and Invisible. New York: The United Nations Children's Fund 2006
16. Houwelling TAJ Ronsmans C Campbell O Kunst AE. Huge-poor-rich inequalities in maternity care: an international comparative study of maternity and child care in developing countries. Bull of the World Health Organization 2007; 85(10): 745-754
17. Van de Poel E Hosseinpoor AR Speybroeck N Ourti TV Vega J. Socioeconomic inequality in malnutrition in developing countries. Bull of the World Health Organization 2007; 86(14): 282-291
18. Egypt Health. Demographic Health Surveys. [http://www.measuredhs.com/countries/country_main.cfm?ctry_id=103 Accessed 2008 Oct 3]
19. Morocco Health. Demographic Health Surveys. [http://www.measuredhs.com/countries/country_main.cfm?ctry_id=27 Accessed 2008 Oct 3]
20. Tunisia Health Demographic Health Surveys. [http://www.measuredhs.com/countries/country_main.cfm?ctry_id=43 Accessed 2008 Oct 3]
21. Hameida J, Billot L, Deschamps JP. Growth of preschool children in the Libyan Arab Jamahiriya: regional and socio-demographic differences. East Mediterr Health J 2002; 8: 13-19
22. Kawaja M Dawns J Meyerson-Knox S Yamout R. Disparities in child health in the Arab region during the 1990s. Int J Equity Health 2009. Available from http://www.equityhealthj.com/content/7/1/24
23. Giashuddin MS Rahman A Rahman F Masshrekey SR Chowdhury M Linnan M Safinaz S. Income Inequality in Child Injury in Bangladesh. Int J Equity Health 2009. Available from http://www.equityhealthj.com/content/pdf/1475-9276-8-7.pdf

CHAPTER 5

Obesity and Diabetes

A. Boutayeb[1,*], S. Mehdad[2], N. Mokhtar[2] and H. Aguenaou[2]

[1] *Laboratoire de Modélisation Stochastique et Déterministe, Mohamed Premier University, Oujda, Morocco, Email: x.boutayeb@menara.ma*

[2] *Unité Mixte de Recherche en Nutrition et Alimentation Unité mixte Université Ibn Tofail, Kenitra-CNESTEN-Rabat, Morocco*

Abstract: Diabetes and obesity currently threaten the health, well-being and economic welfare of virtually every country in the world. Worldwide, overweight and obesity are increasing at alarming rates. As a disease, obesity diminishes both quality of life and life expectancy, but it is also a common risk factor for other diseases like Cardio Vascular Diseases, arthritis, diabetes and many types of cancer. The incidence of diabetes linked to obesity has jumped significantly during the last two decades. Moreover, obesity and type 2-diabetes are affecting people all over the world including children and adolescents. Diabetes and obesity are associated with increased morbidity and mortality in the general population. The twin epidemics constitutes one of the major public health problems challenging all concerned social and economic groups, including scientists, health decision makers, nongovernmental organizations, industry associations, public and private sectors and volunteers.

Keywords: Obesity, overweight, type 2-diabetes, hyperinsulinemia, insulin resistance, adiposity, fat mass, BMI, dietary habits, physical activity.

1. INTRODUCTION

Diabetes and obesity currently threaten the health, well-being and economic welfare of virtually every country in the world. Worldwide [1-4], overweight and obesity are increasing at alarming rates [5-8]. As a disease, obesity diminishes both quality of life and life expectancy, but it is also a common risk factor for other diseases like Cardio Vascular Diseases, arthritis, diabetes and many types of cancer [8-10]. The incidence of diabetes linked to obesity has jumped significantly during the last two decades. Moreover, obesity and type 2-diabetes are affecting people all over the world including children and adolescents. Diabetes and obesity are associated with increased morbidity and mortality in the general population. The twin epidemics constitutes one of the major public health problems challenging all concerned social and economic groups, including scientists, health decision makers, nongovernmental organizations, industry associations, public and private sectors and volunteers. Mathematical models have been used for the dynamics of insulin and glucose [11-14]. We have previously dedicated several publications to different aspects of diabetes and the burden of its complications [15-20]. In the present chapter we deal with the twin epidemic of diabetes and obesity, coined by some authors "diabesity".

2. DIABETES: A SILENT EPIDEMICS

The statistics released by the World Health Organization and the International Diabetes Federation are alarming [1]. The number of diabetes in the world is expected to increase from 194 Million in 2003 to 330 in 2030 with three in four living in developing countries. Moreover, in developed countries most people with diabetes are above the age of retirement, whereas in developing countries those most frequently affected are aged between 35 and 64 which makes the burden heavier in poorer countries. Indeed, in some countries of the Middle East, one in four deaths in adults aged between 35 and 64 years is attributable to diabetes (Table **1**).

---

*Corresponding author

Boutayeb A. (Ed.)

Table 1. Prevalence of diabetes Mellitus in Arab countries (Percent of population age 20 and above)

Country	Rate	Country	Rate
Bahrain	11.0 %	Qatar	15.0 %
Egypt	08.0 %	Saudi Arabia	17.0 %
Iraq	08.6 %	Syria	09.1 %
Kuwait	15.7 %	Tunisia	05.5 %
Morocco	06.6 %	United Arab Emirates	19.6 %
Oman	11.6 %		

The burden is exacerbated by the complications such as blindness, amputations and kidney failure for which diabetes is the leading cause, and the interfering action of Cardio Vascular Diseases (CVDs) which are responsible for between 50 and 80% of deaths in people with diabetes. The burden of premature death from diabetes is similar to that of HIV/AIDS, yet the problem is largely unrecognised [1,2]. It is estimated however, that worldwide, about 50% of diabetic people ignore that they have the disease. This feature worsens the situation especially in developing countries where the delayed diagnosis of diabetes is often associated with onset of complications leading to kidney failure, amputations, retinopathy and cardiovascular problems in general. But the problem is not specific to low-income countries since, for instance, in the United States, there are an estimated 23.6 million people who have type 2 diabetes but around 5.7 million people are ignorant of the disease condition.

Studies in different countries have shown that diabetes is a costly disease accounting for between 2.5 and 15% of the total healthcare expenditure. For the age category 20-79, the world annual direct cost is estimated to be over $153 billion and expected to double in 2025.

According to the National Institute of Diabetes and Digestive Kidney Disease (NIDDK) and the American Diabetes Association, diabetes was the sixth leading cause of death in 1999 with a direct cost of $44 billion and an indirect cost of $54 billion annually. In 2002, the direct and indirect cost totalled $132 billion.

Providing industry and investors with a comprehensive overview of the market in the medium term a strategic report putting the spotlight on current and future drugs that will be used in the treatment of Type I and Type II diabetes was launched with an interesting analysis of diabetes prevalence and trends worldwide, plus current treatment options [21]. According to this report, in 2005, an estimated 1.1 million people around the world died directly from diabetes and more generally, diabetes related causes account for 3.8 million deaths each year. This report gives also striking figures on the economic impact of diabetes. Indeed, it is estimated that the prevention and treatment of diabetes and its complications cost around US$232 billion in 2007 and that by 2025, the cost is likely to exceed US$302.5 billion. In the US, the total economic cost of diabetes was estimated to be US$174 billion in 2007, of which US$116 billion was medical expenditure; US$27 billion was for diabetes care, US$58 billion was for chronic complications related to diabetes, and US$31 billion was attributed to general medical costs. In the UK, around 10% of the NHS budget is spent on treating diabetes and its complications. This equates to around £9 billion (US$16.2 billion). In Japan, general medical expenditure on diabetes amounted to ¥1,116.5 billion (US$10.7 billion) in 2005.

3. OBESITY: AN IRREFUTABLE RISK FACTOR FOR TYPE 2 DIABETES

Type 2 diabetes associated with obesity, coined by some authors 'diabesity', is today the most common form of type 2 diabetes. It is also associated with a number of other cardiovascular risk factors, which constitute the metabolic syndrome [22].

Diabetes and obesity currently threaten the health, well-being and economic welfare of virtually every country in the world. Diabetes and obesity are associated with increased morbidity and mortality in the general population [23]. The increase in the prevalence of type 2 diabetes is closely linked to the upsurge in obesity. About 90% of type 2 diabetes is attributable to excess weight. About 18 million people die every year from cardiovascular disease, for which diabetes and hypertension are major predisposing factors. Propelling the upsurge in cases of diabetes and hypertension is the growing prevalence of overweight and obesity [24]

The World Health Organisation (WHO) defines obesity as'' a condition of abnormal or excessive fat accumulation in adipose tissue, to the extent that health may be impaired''. The body fat being difficult to evaluate directly, a convenient measurement of obesity is given by the Body Mass Index (BMI) which is a simple weight to height ratio (kg/m^2). Accordingly, obesity in adults is defined as a BMI greater than 30 kg/m^2 and international standards for classifying overweight and obesity worldwide are given (Table **2**). In children and adolescent, health professionals often use a BMI "growth chart" or BMI-for-age.

Table 2. Classification of overweight in adults according to BMI

Classification	BMI(kg/m^2)	Risk of co-morbidities
Underweight	<18.5	Low (but risk of other clinical problems increased)
Normal range	18.5 – 24.9	Average
Overweight	>25	
Pre-obese	25-29.9	Increased
Obese class I	30 – 34.9	Moderate
Obese class II	35 – 39.9	Severe
Obese class III	>40	Very severe

However, it should be stressed that BMI may miss some aspects of obesity like the regional distribution of excess body fat in general and excessive abdominal fat in particular. The last form, known as central obesity, is more indicated as a risk for type 2 diabetes.

Worldwide, overweight and obesity affect 1.2 billion of which 300 million are clinically obese. In some developed countries like the USA, the prevalence reaches 60%. But developing countries like those of the Middle East have also a very high prevalence. There is especially two features that need serious reflection: the first one is a concern about the growing prevalence of obesity in children since it is estimated that 10% of the world's children are overweight or obese; the second is the fact that many developing countries are now facing the coexistence of under- and overweight people.

The last two decades have seen a dramatic increase in overweight and obesity rates all over the world, although with some differences intra and inter countries. This alarming trend is linked to a number of factors, including genetic, gender and socio-economic status. Many transition forms (epidemiological, democratic, demographic, ..) have been suspected but the most established link is with the transition from a rural to an urban lifestyle and its corollary of nutrition transition characterised by a higher energy density diet with a greater role for fat and added sugar in foods, greater saturated fat intake mostly from animal sources (Table **3**), reduced intakes of complex carbohydrates and fibres, and reduced fruit and vegetables; with a decrease in physical activity.

Table 3. Trends in dietary supply of fat (grams per capita per day)

Region	1967/69	1977/79	1987/99	1997/99	Change(%) 1967/69-1997/99
World	52.50	57.15	66.60	73.57	21.07
North Africa	43.97	58.43	65.23	63.93	**19.96**
Sub-Saharan Africa	41.47	43.03	41.33	44.47	3.00
East &South-East Asia	27.77	32.27	43.90	51.93	24.16
South Asia	29.07	32.37	38.86	45.53	16.46
China	23.23	27.13	47.53	78.50	55.27
Near East	51.20	62.10	73.50	80.63	**29.43**
Latin America & Caribbean	54.00	64.87	73.40	80.63	26.63
North America	116.90	124.93	138.30	143.00	26.10
European Union	117.20	127.93	142.80	149.03	31.83
Oceania	101.57	101.97	112.83	110.67	9.10
Eastern Europe	90.47	110.53	116.00	104.67	14.20

Classified as a disease, obesity diminishes both quality of life and life expectancy, but it is also a common risk factor for other diseases like CVDs, arthritis, type 2 diabetes and many types of cancer. According to the International Obesity Task Force (IOTF) and the WHO World Health report 2002[3], about 60% of diabetes globally can be attributable to overweight and obesity

4. OBESITY AND INSULIN RESISTANCE

Overweight and Obesity lead to adverse metabolic changes such as insulin resistance, increasing blood pressure and cholesterol [3].

Obesity has been strongly associated with insulin resistance in normoglycaemic persons and in individuals with type 2 diabetes [25]. It plays a central role in the insulin resistance syndrome, which includes hyperinsulinemia, hypertension, hyperlipidemia, type 2 diabetes mellitus [26,27], and an increased risk of atherosclerotic cardiovascular disease [28,29].

Resistance of the body to the actions of insulin results in increased production of this hormone by the pancreas and ensuing hyperinsulinemia. Obesity beginning in childhood often precedes the hyperinsulinemic state [30,31],

The association of obesity with the insulin resistance syndrome is not only related to the degree of obesity but also seems to be critically dependent on body fat distribution. Thus, individuals with greater degrees of central adiposity develop this syndrome more frequently than do those with a peripheral body fat distribution. [32], The increased prevalence of excessive visceral obesity is closely associated with rising incidence of cardiovascular diseases and type 2 diabetes mellitus [32]. Such association between adiposity and insulin resistance has been reported in adults and children [34,35].

On the other hand, body fat mass distribution and deposition are determined by multiple environmental and genetic factors. [36,37]. Moreover, insulin has anabolic effects on fat metabolism leading to fat deposition and obesity [38].

So several mechanisms whereby insulin resistance could cause an alteration in lipid metabolism have been described. Hyperinsulinemia is known to enhance hepatic very-low-density lipoprotein synthesis and thus may directly contribute to the increased plasma triglyceride and LDL cholesterol levels. Resistance to the action of insulin on lipoprotein lipase in peripheral tissues may also contribute to elevated triglyceride and LDL cholesterol levels. [39,40]

Adipocyte-specific or -enriched hormones are now known as adipokines and are often actively involved in the regulation of diverse physiologic functions such as energy homeostasis, insulin sensitivity, inflammation, appetite, angiogenesis, and blood pressure. Obesity is a common underlying condition for cardiovascular diseases and coexists with insulin resistance caused by the accumulated adipose tissue [41,42]

Obesity and dietary habits are the principal risk factors for diabetes of type 2. It is estimated that up to 80% of cases of coronary heart disease, and up to 90% of cases of types 2 diabetes, could potentially be avoided through changing lifestyle factors. [2, 26-28]:

5. HEALTH EQUITY AND "DIABESITY"

In the foreword to the WHO Report 2003, the WHO Director-General wrote: "Two of the most striking findings in this report are to be found almost side by side. One is that in poor countries today there   are 170 million underweight children, over three million of whom will die this year as a result. The other is that there are more than one billion adults wordwide who are overweight and at least 300 million who are clinically obese. Among these, about half a million people in North America and Western Europe combined will have died this year from obesity-related diseases....Could the contrast between the haves and have-nots ever be more starkly illustrated?"[43].

Lifestyles constitute a social determinant underlying health inequity. Between and within countries, there are social differences in diets and physical activity. In almost all countries, independently of their level of economic development, people from lower socio-economic groups have less healthy diet than people from higher socio-economic groups. Worldwide and in low-income countries in particular, millions of people survive on less than one dollar a day. Consequently, their main concern is about the minimum of food that protects them from starving. In these conditions, talking about healthy diet is a non sense!

Healthy diet in general and consumption of fruit and vegetable in particular, varies according to the level of income as indicated by a recent report devoted to a critical analysis of public health policies in eight European countries [44]. This report indicates that in England, nearly 40% of women from the highest income quintile were eating 5 or more portions of fruit and vegetables per day compared to less than 20% of women in the lowest income quintile

In Sweden, only 5% of men and 14 of women aged 18-84 years reported that they ate the equivalent of 500 grams of fruit/vegetables per day in 2006, around 1/3 of all adults exercise less than the recommended amount of 30muniutes per day and 14% of the population reported being sedentary in their spare time. However, sedentary lifestyle was more common for those who have not attained an upper secondary education and eating habits were seen to vary between different cultural and social backgrounds

6. DISCUSSION

By reducing insulin sensitivity and increasing insulin resistance, obesity/overweight constitutes a barrier to the mechanism transforming food and glucose to energy. In the presence of obesity, a vicious cycle is set off: the quantity of insulin released is not sufficient to convert adequately food into energy. Consequently, there is more demand on pancreatic production of insulin, which leads to hyperinsulinemia which in turn increases the need to eat, and the final result is often type 2-diabetes.

This vicious cycle also explains why people cannot loose fat even with diet strategies [20].

As a conclusion, prevention remains the best remedy against excess weight and its devastating consequences from cardiovascular diseases, diabetes, cancer and other non communicable diseases.

The main strategies for prevention and treatment of overweight and obesity, which need to involve community, school and family, are the promotion of lifestyle interventions, including as a correct dietary approach, rich in fruit and vegetables and low-fat dairy products, and physical activity [45]. Nevertheless, interventions are needed to improve physical activity and diet in communities nationwide. Thus, it's recommended to eat fewer calories and increase physical activity to more than 150 min/wk [46].

There is evidence that regular physical activity is beneficial for a range of health outcomes, including improved blood lipid profiles, blood pressure, body composition, glucose metabolism, bone strength and psychological health [47] On the other hand, weight loss is associated with a decrease in insulin concentration and an increase in insulin sensitivity in adults [48] and adolescents [4,50].

7. ACKNOWLEDGEMENTS

8. REFERENCES

1. WHO-IDF. Diabetes:. Action Now.[http://www.who]
2. Boutayeb A, Boutayeb S. The burden of non communicable diseases in developing countries. International Journal on Equity in Health 2005 doi:10.1186/1475-9276-5-1
3. WHO. Diet, Nutrition and the prevention of chronic diseases. WHO Technical report Series 916, Geneva, World Health Organization 2003.
4. WHO report 2002. Reducing Risk: Promoting Life., Geneva, World Health Organization 2002
5. WHO. Obesity: preventing and managing the global epidemic. WHO Technical report Series 894. Geneva, World Health Organization, 2000
6. Drewnowski A, Popkin BM. The nutrition transition: new trends in the global diet. Nutrition Reviews 1997; 55: 31-43
7. Barbara B. Kahn and Jeffrey S. Flier: Obesity and insulin resistance. The Journal of Clinical Investigation 2000; 106: 473-481.
8. James P.T et al. The Worldwide Obesity Epidemic. OBESITY RESEARCH 2001; 9(4):228S-233S.
9. Sjostrand M, Holmang A, Strindberg L and Lonnroth P. Estimation of muscle interstitial insulin, glucose, and lactat in type 2 diabetic subjects. Am J Physiol Endocrinol Metab 2000; 279: 1097-1103.
10. Sjostrand M, Gudbjornsdottir S, Strindberg L and Lonnroth P. Delayed Transcapillary Delivery of Insulin to Muscle Interstitial Fluid After Oral Glucose Load in Obese Subjects. Diabetes 2005; 54:152-157.
11. Bellazi R, Nucci G, Cobelli C. The subcutaneous route to insulin-dependent diabetes theory. Review. IEEE Engineering in Medicine and Biology 2001; 20:56-64
12. Parker RS, Doyle FJ, Peppas NA. The intravenous route to the blood glucose control. Review. IEEE Engineering in Medicine and Biology 2001; 24:65-73
13. Bergman RN, Ider YZ, Bowden CR & Cobelli C: Quantitative estimation of insulin sensitivity. Am. J. Physiol. 1979; 236:E667-E677.
14. De Gaetano A, Arino O. Mathematical modelling of the Intra- Venous Glucose Tolerance Test. J Math Biol 2000; 40:136-168.
15. Boutayeb A, Kerfati A . Mathematical models in diabetology. Measurement and Control, C, AMSE 1994; 44: 53-63
16. Boutayeb A, Derouich M. Age structured models for diabetes in East Morocco. Mathematics and Computers in Simulation 2002; 58: 215-229.
17. Boutayeb A, Chetouani A. Dynamics of a disabled population in Morocco. BioMedical Engineering Online 2003 doi:10.1186/1475-925X-2-2 [http://www.biomedical-engineering-online.com/content/2/1/2]
18. Boutayeb A, Twizell EH. An age structured model for complications of diabetes mellitus in Morocco. Simulation Modelling Practice and Theory 2004; 12: 77-78
19. Boutayeb A, Twizell EH, Achouyab K, Chetouani A. A mathematical model for the burden of diabetes and its complications. BioMedical Engineering Online 2004 doi:10.1186/1475-925X-3-20 [http://www.biomedical-engineering-online.com/content/3/1/20]
20. Derouich M, Boutayeb A. The effect of physical exercise on the dynamics of glucose and insulin. Journal of Biomechanics 2002; 35: 911-917.
21. [http://www.researchandmarkets.com/product/c73c12/diabetes_drug_discoveries_2009_what_the_futur].

22.   Yki-Yarvinen H. Toxicity of hyperglycaemia in type 2 diabetes. Diabetes Metab Rev. 1998;14 Suppl 1:S45-S50.
23.   A. H. Barnett, Sudhesh Kumar. Obesity and Diabetes (eBook). *Circulation.* 2003;107:1448
24.   Must A, Spadano J, Coakley EH, Field AE, Colditz G, Dietz WH. The disease burden associated with overweight and obesity. Jama 1999 ; 282(16):1523-1529.
25.   Parvez H et al. Obesity and Diabetes in the Developing World - A Growing Challenge. N Eng J Med. 2007; 356(3): 213-215
26.   Bonadonna RC, Groop L, Kraemer N, et al. Obesity and insulin resistance in humans: a dose-response study. Metabolism. 1990; 39: 452–459.
27.   Després JP. Visceral obesity, insulin resistance, and dyslipidemia: contribution of endurance exercise training to the treatment of the plurimetabolic syndrome. Exerc Sport Sci Rev. 1997; 25:271-300
28.   Bouchard C, Shephard RJ, Stephens TE. Physical Activity Fitness, and Health: Second International Consensus Symposium, May 1992. Champaign, Ill: Human Kinetics Publishers; 1994.
29.   Pinhas-Hamiel O, Dolan LM, Daniels SR, et al. Increased incidence of non-insulin-dependent diabetes mellitus among adolescents. J Pediatr. 1996; 128:608–615.
30.   Fagot-Campagna A, Pettitt DJ, Engelgau MM, et al. Type 2 diabetes among North American children and adolescents: an epidemiologic review and a public health perspective. J Pediatr. 2000; 136: 664–672.
31.   Steinberger J, Moorehead C, Katch V, et al. Relationship between insulin resistance and abnormal lipid profile in obese adolescents. J Pediatr. 1995; 126: 690–695.
32.   Sinaiko AR, Jacobs DR Jr, Steinberger J, et al. Insulin resistance syndrome in childhood: associations of the euglycemic insulin clamp and fasting insulin with fatness and other risk factors. J Pediatr. 2001; 139: 700–707.
33.   Kissebah AH, Krakower GR. Regional adiposity and morbidity. Physiol Rev. 1994; 74: 761–811.
34.   Hajer, G.R., Van Haeften, T.W., Visseren, F.L.J. Adipose tissue dysfunction in obesity, diabetes, and vascular diseases. European Heart Journal 2008; 29(24):2959-2971
35.   Arslanian S, Suprasongsin C. Insulin sensitivity, lipids, and body composition in childhood: is "syndrome X" present? J Clin Endocrinol Metab. 1996; 81:1058–1062.
36.   Caprio S, Bronson M, Sherwin RS, et al. Co-existence of severe insulin resistance and hyperinsulinaemia in pre-adolescent obese children. Diabetologia. 1996; 39:1489-1497.
37.   Ford ES, Williamson DF, Liu S: Weight change and diabetes incidence: findings from a national cohort of US adults. Am J Epidemiol 1997; 146(3):214-222.
38.   Resnick HE, Valsania P, Halter JB, Lin X. Relation of weight gain and weight loss on subsequent diabetes risk in overweight adults. Journal of epidemiology and community health 2000; 54(8):596-602.
39.   Nora Franceschini et al. Diabetes-specific genetic effects on obesity traits in American Indian populations: the Strong Heart Family Study. BMC Medical Genetics 2008, 9:90doi:10.1186/1471-2350-9-90
40.   Pykalisto OJ, Smith PH, Brunzell JD. Determinants of human adipose tissue lipoprotein lipase: effect of diabetes and obesity on basal- and diet-induced activity. J Clin Invest. 1975; 56: 1108–1117.
41.   Sadur CN, Yost TJ, Eckel RH. Insulin responsiveness of adipose tissue lipoprotein lipase is delayed but preserved in obesity. J Clin Endocrinol Metab. 1984; 59 : 1176-1182.
42.   Grundy SM. Hypertriglyceridemia, insulin resistance, and the metabolic syndrome. Am J Cardiol 1999; 83:25-29.
43.   The World Health Report 2003. Shaping the Future. World Health Organization, Geneva, 2003
44.   Hogsted C, Moberg H, uLundgren B, Backhans M. Health for all? A critical analysis of public health polices in eight European countries. Swedish National Institute of Public Health, 2009.
45.   T. Nakamura, K. Tokunaga and I. Shimomura et al., Contribution of visceral fat accumulation to the development of coronary artery disease in non-obese men, Atheroscrerosis 1994; 107:239-246.
46.   Virdis, A., Ghiadoni, S., Masi, S., Versari, D., Daghini, E., Giannarelli, C., Salvetti, A., Taddei, S. Obesity in the childhood: A link to adult hypertension. Current Pharmaceutical Design 2009; 15(10):1063-1071
47.   Ali H. Mokdad et al. The Continuing Epidemics of Obesity and Diabetes in the United States JAMA. 2001; 286:1195-1200.
48.   Strong WB, Malina RM, Blimkie CJR, et al. Evidence-based physical activity for school-age youth. J Pediatr 2005;146:732–7.
49.   Su HY, Sheu WH, Chin HM, et al. Effect of weight loss on blood pressure and insulin resistance in normotensive and hypertensive obese individuals. Am J Hypertens. 1995; 8: 1067–1071.
50.   Rocchini AP, Katch V, Schork A, et al. Insulin and blood pressure during weight loss in obese adolescents. Hypertension. 1987; 10: 267–273.

56   *Social Determinants, Health Equity And Human Development, 2009, 56-61*

CHAPTER 6

Modelling for the Dynamics and the Burden of Dengue: A Review

Mohammed Derouich[1,2] and Abdesslam Boutayeb[1,*]

[1]*Department of Mathematics Faculty of Sciences, Boulevard Mohamed VI, BP: 717 Oujda, Morocco, Email: x.boutayeb@menara.ma,* [2]*Email: derouichm@yahoo.fr*

Abstract: Among the re-emergent diseases, dengue fever/dengue haemorrhagic fever is one of the most important by its wide spreading, the frequency of its epidemics and the complexity caused by the four virus serotypes associated with it. With more than 2.5 billion at risk, the global burden of dengue is growing dramatically. The literature associated with different aspects of dengue is abundant, this paper is a review of a large part of publications dealing with dengue and environmental health, the burden of disease and mathematical modelling mainly during the last decade.

Keywords: Dengue, mathematical models, haemorrhagic fever, environmental health, burden of disease.

1. INTRODUCTION

Infectious diseases were the main causes of death during the last millennium. Life expectancy was often limited by recurrent uncontrolled epidemics. After the Second World War, with medical research achievements in terms of vaccination, antibiotics and improvement of life conditions, it was expected that infectious diseases were going to disappear. Consequently, in developed countries the efforts have been concentrated on Non Communicable Diseases (NCDs) such as Cardio Vascular Diseases (CVDs) and cancer. However, at the dawn of the third millennium, the world population is facing a double burden of NCDs and infectious diseases. Non Communicable Diseases, once known as the disease of "the rich", are now sweeping the entire globe with the main part of the increasing trend attributable to developing countries where CVDs, cancer and diabetes are flourishing [1-5]. The socio economic transition engaged by medium income countries is believed to be the responsible of this evolution. But, at the same time, infectious diseases continue to be the major causes of mortality and morbidity in developing countries. Well known existing, emerging and re-emerging diseases like tuberculosis, cholera, meningitis, hepatitis, malaria, dengue, yellow fever, AIDS, Ebola, SARS and others are causing suffering and mortality to a wide population in the developing world but developed countries are also at risk [6-8]. Measured in terms of numbers of deaths and Disability Adjusted Life Years (DALYs) (which is a combination of Years Lived with Disability(YLD) and Years of Life Lost from premature death(YLL) [9], the burden of these diseases is alarming and calls for urgent actions and efficient strategies. If the present trend is maintained, developing countries, with poor budgets and ill-health systems will not be able to cope with the double burden of infective and non infective diseases (Table **1**).

Table 1. The burden of risk factors

Risk factor	DALYs (1990)(7)	% of total DALYs	DALYs (2000)(1)	% of total DALYs
Underweight	220	15.9	138	9.5
Poor water, hygiene, sanitation	93	06.8	54	3.7
Unsafe sex	49	03.5	92	6.3
Alcohol	48	03.5	58	4
Occupation	38	02.7	23	1.6
Tobacco	36	02.6	59	4.1
Blood pressure	19	01.4	64	4.5
Physical inactivity	14	01.0	27	1.9
Illicit drugs	8	00.6	11	0.7
Air pollution	7	00.5	19	1.3

*Corresponding author

Low and medium income countries must abandon considering health and education as non productive sectors. In contrary, it is now proved and commonly admitted that good health and education are prerequisites for economic development and especially for sustainable development [10, 11].

Among the infectious diseases, dengue fever, especially known in Southeast Asia, is now endemic in more than 100 countries world-wide. Its incidence has increased fourfold since 1970 and nearly half the world population (2.5-3 billion) is now at risk. In 1998, 1.2 million cases were reported to WHO in 56 countries. It estimated that more than 50 million people are infected every year of which half a million of DHF [12].

The two recognised species of the vector transmitting dengue are Aedes aegypti and Aedes albopictus. The first is highly anthropophilic, thriving in crowded cities and biting primarily during the day while the later is less anthropophilic and inhabits rural areas.

Consequently, the importance of dengue is two- fold: (i) With increasing urbanisation, crowded cities, poor sanitation and lack of hygiene, environmental conditions foster the spread of the disease which, even in the absence of fatal forms, breeds significant economic and social costs(absenteeism, immobilisation, debilitation, medication). (ii) The potential risk of evolution towards the haemorrhagic form and the dengue shock syndrome with high economic costs and which may lead to death. In the two cases, the burden of disease can be measured in terms of DALYs.

Dengue fever illustrates clearly the links between health and sustainable development. Any tentative to predict the epidemics and prevent the disasters caused by the disease will impose a global strategy that takes into account environmental conditions, levels of poverty and illiteracy and eventually, degree of coverage by vaccination programs.

It is thus important to consider an overview which incorporates global analysis of the burden and cost-effective strategies, with special attention to epidemiological studies and interdisciplinary research.

For better understanding of the disease dynamics, there is a need to diagnose all the parameters and their effect (geographic, economic, social, biologic). To this aim, data should be gathered, organised and analysed and consequent strategies can be formulated and again tested and evaluated. Weekly epidemiological record, Dengue bulletin and DengueNet constitute interesting tools but there is still a long way to go in order to overcome unreported and underestimated situations. Indeed, according to a prospective study conducted recently in north-east Brazil, the authors estimated that around 560000 individuals were infected by one or two serotypes of dengue, whereas the official system of notification had recorded only 360 cases [13]. Concrete multivariable data will also allow for better development of mathematical models, computer software and biomedical issues.

Mathematical models have known an extraordinary development since the model proposed in 1760 by Bernoulli on smallpox and variolation. With the advantages of computing and simulation, they offered alternative and complementary methods for the analysis and the comprehension of many diseases. Deterministic and stochastic models provide interesting tools in order to formulate different scenarios, test strategies, evaluate cost effective decisions, and forecast trends. They also allow for the control of variables and parameters and may prevent from costly and dangerous operations. A huge number of books, papers and reviews have dealt with different aspects of mathematical modelling and infectious diseases [14-23]. In particular, an exhaustive list of publications can be found in the review by Hethcote [24].

2. DENGUE AND ENVIRONMENT

Principles 1 and 5 of the Rio Declaration stipulate respectively that: "humans are at the centre of concerns for sustainable development. They are entitled to a healthy and productive life in harmony with nature" and "eradicating poverty is an indispensable requirement for sustainable development, in order to decrease the disparities in standards of living and better meet the needs of the majority of the people of the world". Accordingly, many recent publications have dealt with sustainable development, global environment and public health [11], Environmental health and disease control [25], Linking environment and health and characterising environmental hazards [26], environmental health [27], Sustainable Development in a Dynamic World [28].

According to the Scientific Working Group on Dengue (SWG) [29], the environmental and social determinants of dengue transmission risks will continue to expand in the coming years and the increasing threat of dengue necessitates the adoption of a multi-prolonged approach which takes into account the changing social and environmental conditions.

The growing burden caused by Tobacco and its high correlation with many chronic diseases such as cancer and CVDs is well established but it is interesting to see how smoking can also foster diseases like dengue fever through deforestation especially in developing countries [10].

3. THE BURDEN OF DF/DHF: A GLOBAL HEALTH PROBLEM

The re-emergence of dengue and its wide spreading during the last few decades constitute a major problem for the World Health Organisation and health authorities in developing countries in particular. With more than 2.5 billion people at risk, the disease is necessitating large effort for the comprehension of its dynamics, the evaluation of its impact and the search for means of control. Many authors have presented the disease as a major health problem either for the last decades of the 20th century or for the third millennium [30-39]. The need for research and surveillance is often dealt with and many authors have stressed that DF/DHF is still perceived as unimportant and receives little attention despite its social and economic impact being similar to some of the most visible infectious diseases. Without being exhaustive we can refer to [40,41].

In [40] the economic impact of dengue in Puerto Rico was assessed using Disability-Adjusted Life Years over the decade 1984-1994. According to the authors, dengue caused an average of 658 DALYs per year per million population with a maximum estimate for 1994 of 2153 DALYs/million population. The loss to dengue is similar to the losses per million population in the Latin American and Caribbean region attributed to any one of the following diseases or disease clusters: the child cluster (polio, measles, pertussis, diphtheria, tetanus), meningitis, hepatitis or malaria. The loss is also of the same order of magnitude as any one of the following: tuberculosis, sexually transmitted diseases (excluding AIDS), tropical cluster chagas, leishmanisis) or intestinal helminths.

In [41], the evolution of the disease was considered through three dates: 1930, 1970 and 2001.The author recalls the successful Ae.aegypti control program in the 1950s and 1960s. Estimation of cost were given for different periods and countries: Puerto Rico (1977 & 1994), Cuba (1981), Thailand (2002). Unreported indirect costs such as productivity and time away from work and school and other social costs occurring during inter-epidemics periods can be taken into account in terms of DALYs. Accordingly, DF/DHF is seen to have a total impact of the same order of magnitude as many of the major infectious diseases such as malaria, tuberculosis, hepatitis, bacterial meningitis and others.

Global DALYs scores were also used to compare rabies and other selected diseases [42]. This study indicated that dengue was responsible for 653000DALYS in 2001.

Other estimations of deaths, costs of DF/DHF and global burden using DALYs for different countries are given in [43]

Finally, among the dengue control strategies, vaccination is the most promising. So far, the difficulties in elaborating a vaccine stemmed from the fact that the vaccine must protect against the four serotypes at the same time. Research is encouraged, supported by cost-effective analysis in order to produce a vaccine in the very short term.

The Cost-effectiveness of a paediatric dengue vaccine was discussed through a model of vaccinating children at 15 months in Southeast Asia. The economic feasibility of a paediatric tetravalent vaccine was ascertained by comparing the gross and net cost per 1000 population (of all ages) with the cost per DALY saved. According to the author's conclusion, the potential vaccine would be highly cost-effective [44]. Other publication dealt with the importance of vaccination in the control of dengue disease [45-47].

4. MODELLING, EPIDEMIOLOGY AND SURVEILLANCE

Different mathematical models were proposed. In general, they use compartmental dynamics with Susceptible, Exposed, Infective and Removed for human; and Susceptible and Infective for mosquito.

Beside the references cited in the introduction, some models formulated for infectious diseases transmitted by vectors (Malaria, Chagas,…) can be directly or indirectly of interest for dengue modelling [48-53].

SEIRS models were considered in [54] with an evaluation of the impact of ultra-low volume (ULV) insecticide applications on dengue epidemics. The values of basis parameters used in simulation by the authors constituted a data source (table 2) for other authors.

Table 2. Basic parameters (53)

Name of the parameter	Value
Transmission probability of vector to human	0.75
Transmission probability of human to vector	0.75
Bites per susceptible mosquito per day	0.50
Bites per infectious mosquito per day	1.00
Effective contact rate, human to vector	0.375
Effective contact rate, vector to human	0.75
Birth rate of human population	0.00015
Human life span	25000 days(68.5years)
Vector life span	4 days
Host infection duration	3 days

In the dissertation of Esteva under the supervision of Varga [55] four chapters were dedicated to the dynamics of dengue disease. In the first chapter, a general model with the population of susceptible and infectious human assumed constant and facing only one virus.

In the second chapter, the human population was supposed to grow exponentially and to have a constant disease rate.

The chapter three dealt with two serotypes of virus and variable human population, whereas the last chapter analysed the impact of vertical transmission and interrupted feeding on the dynamics of the disease.

The basic reproductive number P_0 was estimated from serological data for 25 states of Mexico. Comparison was made with other published results. It was found that coexistence of two serotypes is possible for a large range of parameters. The results were also published in four papers [56-59].

In [60], considering competitive exclusion of one of the strains as a result of the interaction, the authors argue that the existence of this phenomenon is the product of the interaction between a super-infection process and frequency-dependent host contact rates.

While pointing out that the idea of two viruses coexisting in the same epidemic is controversial, a mathematical model with two different viruses acting at separated intervals of time was discussed in [61,62]. Simulations with different values of the parameters were performed and vaccination strategies were discussed.

Assuming that dengue epidemics are strongly influenced by the amount of rainfall amongst other environmental factors, a model with varying vector population was considered in [63]

According to the Report of the Scientific Working Group on Insect and Human Health [64)], the sequencing of the entire Aedes aegypti genome, anticipated to be completed by 2004, will open an unparalleled opportunity to explore the interaction of dengue viruses with the vector.

The report indicates how modelling with bioinformatics will provide research with interesting tools.

The number of publications dealing with dengue is growing exponentially and it is not our intention to give an exhaustive list. More references can be found in [65-67] and especially in the review by and Kuno [68] and Gubler [69].

Finally, it is worth pointing out that, during the last decade many activities have been organised in order to foster epidemiological studies, understand the dynamics of dengue and discuss strategies for management and control of dengue and dengue haemorrhagic. The activities varied from academic research discussions (ICTP-Mathematical ecology group, IMA workshop, IRD seminar, Pacific Institute workshop) , professional organisations directives (WHO, SERARO, PAHO, TDR) and field actions from regional authorities

5. CONCLUSION

Dengue/dengue haemorrhagic fever has become a major health problem, its burden is afflicting many developing countries but the disease may emerge also in developed countries if the present trend is not stopped. By the complexity of the serotypes, the socio-economic and environmental conditions characterizing this disease and its spreading, a huge number of studies are published on different aspects of dengue. In this paper, without being exhaustive, we reviewed some of the papers dealing with dengue and environment, the burden of disease and modelling. We made some comparisons between results of different authors and tried to present the problem of dengue in its global dimension

6. REFERENCES

1. WHO. Shaping the Future. The world Health Report 2003, WHO, Geneva, 2003
2. WHO. Diet, nutrition and the prevention of Chronic diseases. WHO technical report Series 916, WHO, Geneva, 2003.
3. WHO - IARC. Biennial Report 2002-2003. IARC, Lyon, France, 2003.
4. Boutayeb A, Twizell EH. An age structured model for complications of diabetes mellitus in Morocco. Simulation Modelling Practice and Theory 2004; 12: 77-78
5. Parkin DM, Pisani P and Ferlay J. Global Cancer Statistics. CA CANCER J CLIN, 1999, 49 : 33 - 64
6. Fourth Intergovernmental Preparatory Meeting. Health and the environment in the WHO European Region: Situation and Policy at the beginning of the 21st Century, WHO Regional Office for Europe, Copenhagen, 2004.
7. Murray CJL, Lopez AD, eds. The global burden of disease: a comprehensive assessment of mortality and disability from diseases, injuries and risk factors in 1990 and projected to 2020. Global Burden of Disease and Injury, Vol 1. Harvard School of Public Health on behalf of WHO, Cambridge, MA, 1996.
8. Rodhain F. Impacts sur la santé: le cas des maladies à vecteurs, Institut Pasteur, 2004
9. Mathers CD, Bernard C, Iburg KM, Inoue M, Fat DM, Shibuya K, Stein C, Tomijima N, Xu H. Global Burden of Disease in 2002: data sources, methods and results. Global Programme on Evidence for Health Policy Discussion Paper N0.54, WHO, 2003.
10. WHO. Tobacco & Health in the Developing World: A background Paper for the High Level Round Table on Tobacco Control and Development Policy, Brussels, 2003.
11. McMichael AJ and Kjellstrom T. Sustainable Development, Global Environmental Change and Public Health. ISUMA, 2002, ISSN 1492-0611.
12. DengueNet: [http/www.who.int/dengue]
13. Teixeira MG, Barretoo ML, Costa MCN, Ferreira LDA, Vasconcelos PFC and Cairncross S. Dynamics of dengue virus circulation: a silent epidemic in a complex urban area. Trop. Med. Intern. Health, 2002, 7:757-762.
14. Anderson RM and May RM. Infectious Diseases of Humans: Dynamics and Control. Oxford University Press, Oxford, 1992.
15. Bailey NTJ. The mathematical theory of infectious Diseases. Griffin, London, 1975.
16. Boutayeb A, Chetouani A and Derouich M. Eléments d'Analyse Numérique avec Applications aux Modèles Biomathématiques et Ecologiques. Trifa Edition, Berkane, 2003.
17. DeAngelis DL and Gross LJ. Individual-based models and approaches in ecology. Chapman & Hall, 1990.
18. Dieckman O and Heesterbeek J. Mathematical Epidemiology of Infectious Diseases. Wiley, New York, 2000.
19. Hethcote HR. A thousand and one epidemic models. In: frontiers in Levin(ed.), Theoretical biology, Lectures notes in Biomath. 100, Spring-Verlag, Berlin, 1994, 504 -515.
20. Kot M. Elements of mathematical ecology. Cambridge University Press, Cambridge, UK, 2000.
21. Ross R. The prevention of Malaria , 2nd ed., Murray, London, 1911.
22. Hoppensteadt F. Mathematical Theories of Populations: Demographics, Genetics and epidemics. SIAM, Philadelphia, 1975.
23. Wickwire K. Mathematical models for the control of pests and infectious diseases: a survey. Theoret. Population Biol., 1977, 11 : 182 - 238
24. Hethcote HR. The mathematics of infectious diseases, Review. SIAM Review, 2000, 42(4) : 599-653.
25. Anonymous. Dengue Fever: An environmental Plague for the New Millennium? Medical Service Corporation International, Arlington, 2000.
26. World Resources Institute. Characterising Environmental Hazards, 2004 [http/www.wri.org/wr-98-99/001-hzrd.htm]
27. Anonymous. Environmental health. The World Bank www.worldbank.org/hnp
28. The World Bank. Sustainable Development in a Dynamic World. World Development Report 2003, The World Bank, Washington, D.C, 2003.
29. Scientific Working Group On Dengue. Meeting Report, UNPD/World Bank/WHO special Programme for Research and Training in Tropical Diseases(TDR), 2000.
30. Gubler DJ. Dengue. In: Monath T.P.(ed.), The arbovirus: Epidemiologgy and Ecology. CRC Press, Florida, USA, 1986, 213-261
31. Gubler DJ. Dengue and dengue haemorrhagic fever in the Americas. PR Hlth Sci J. 1987, 6:107-111.
32. Gubler DJ. And Casta-Valez A. A Programme for Prevention and Control of Epidemic Dengue and Dengue Haemorrhagic Fever in Puerto Rico and the U.S Virgin Islands. Bull PAHO, 1991, 25:237-247.
33. Gubler DJ and Trent DW. Emergence of epidemic dengue/dengue haemorrhagic fever as a public health problem in the Americas. Infect Agents Dis. , 1994, 2:383-393.
34. Gubler DJ and Clarck GG. Dengue/dengue haemorrhagic fever: The emergence of global health problem . Emerg Infect Dis., 1995, 1:55-57.
35. Gubler DJ. Epidemic Dengue/Dengue Haemorrhagic Fever: A Global Public Health Problem in the 21st Century. Dengue Bulletin, 1997, 1:55-57.
36. Gubler DJ. Dengue and C: Its history and resurgence as a global public health problem. In: Gubler DJ and Kuno G (ed.), Dengue and dengue haemorrhagic fever. CAB International, New York, 1997, 1-22.
37. Gubler DJ and Meltzer M. The impact of dengue/ dengue haemorrhagic fever on the developing world. Adv. Virus Res. , 1999, 53: 35-70.
38. Halstead SB. The XXth century dengue pandemic: need for surveillance and research. World Health Statistics Quarterly, 1992, 45: 292-298.
39. Halstead SB. Epidemiology of dengue and dengue haemorrhagic fever. In: Gubler DJ, Kuno G (eds.), Dengue and dengue haemorrhagic fever. CAB International, New York, NY, 1997, 23-44
40. Meltzer MI, Rigau-Perez JG, Clark GG, Reiter P and Gubler DJ. Using DALY to assess the economic impact of dengue in Puerto Rico: 1984-1994. Am. J. Trop. Med. Hyg., 1998, 59:265-271.
41. Gubler DJ. Epidemic dengue/ dengue haemorrhagic fever as a public health, social and economic problem in the 21st century. TRENDS in microbiology, 2002, 10: 100-103
42. Coleman PG, Fèvre EM, and Cleaveland S. Estimating the Public Health Impact of Rabies. Emerging Infectious Diseases, 2004, 10(1):140-142
43. Strategic Direction Research. Dengue: disease burden and epidemiological trends, 2002, [www.who.int/tdr].
44. Shepard DS, Suaya JA, Halstead SB, Nathan MB, Gubler DJ, Mahoney RT, Wang DNC, Meltzer MI. Cost-effectiveness of a pediatric dengue vaccine. Vaccine, 2004, 22:1275-1280.
45. Shepard DS. Modeling in CE analysis: sensitivity analysis : impact of DHF rates and cost of vaccine on Cost effectiveness [http/www.sihp.brandeis.edu], 2001.
46. WHO. Dengue haemorrhagic fever: Diagnosis, treatment and control, Geneva 1986.
47. Kinney R.M and Huang CYH. Development of new vaccines against dengue fever and Japanese encephalitis. Interviology, 2001, 44: 176-197.

48. Castillo-Chavez C, Huang W and Li J. Competitive exclusion and multiple strains in an SIS STD model. SIAM J. Appl. Math. 1999, 59: 1790-1811.
49. Dietz K. Transmission and control of arbovirus diseases. Proceedings of the Society for Industrial and Applied Mathematics: Epidemiology, Philadelphia, 1974, 104-121.
50. Dietz K. The incidence of infectious diseases under the influence of seasonal fluctuations. In: Berger et al. (eds.), Mathematical Models in Medicine. Lecture Notes in Biomath. 11, Springer-Verlag, Berlin, 1976: 1- 15
51. Dietz K. Epidemiology Interference of Virus Population. J Math Biol , 1979, 8: 291-300.
52. Mena-Lorca J and Hethcote HW. Dynamic models of infectious diseases as a regulators of population sizes. J. Math. Biol. , 1992, 30:693-716
53. Velasco-Henandez JX. A model for Chagas Disease Involving Transmission by Vectors and Blood Transfusion. Theoretical Population Biology, 1994, 46(1): 1-31
54. Newton EA and Reiter A. A model of the transmission of dengue fever with an evaluation of the impact of ultra-low volume (ULV) insecticide applications on dengue epidemics. Am J Trop Med Hyg, 1992, 47: 709-720.
55. Esteva L. Analysis of a dengue disease. PhD. Dissertation, Depto. De Matematicas, CINVESTAV-IPN, Mexico, 1997.
56. Esteva L and Vargas C. Analysis of a dengue disease transmission model. Mathematical Biosciences, 1998, 150(2): 131-151.
57. Esteva L and Vargas C. A model for dengue disease with variable human population. Journal of Mathematical Biology, 1999, 38: 220-240.
58. Esteva L and Vargas C. Influence of vertical and mechanical transmission on the dynamics of dengue disease. Mathematical Biosciences, 2000, 167(1): 51 - 64.
59. Esteva L and Vargas C. Coexistence of different serotypes of dengue virus. Journal of Mathematical Biology, 2003, 46: 31-47.
60. Feng Z. and Vealsco-Hernandez V. Competitive exclusion in a vector-host model for the dengue fever. Journal of Mathematical Biology, 1997, 35: 523-544.
61. Derouich M. Modélisation et simulation de modèles avec et sans structure d'âge: application au diabète et à la fièvre dengue. Ph.D. Facuty of sciences, Oujda, Morocco, 2001.
62. Derouich M, Boutayeb A and Twizell EH. A model of dengue fever. Biomedical Engineering Online, 2003, 2:4.
63. Ang KC and Li Z. Modelling the spread of Dengue in Singapore. Proceeding for the Modelling and Simulation Conference 1999, Vol. 2, New Zeland, 555-560.
64. Report of the Scientific Working Group on Insect Vectors and Human Health. Insect Vectors and Human Health, TDR/SWG/VEC/03.1, Geneva, 2002
65. Soewono E., Supriatna AK. A two-dimensional model for the transmission of dengue fever disease. Bull. Malays. Math. Sci., 2001, 24(2), 49-57.
66. WHO. Dengue Haemorrhagic Fever: Diagnosis, treatment, Prevention and Control, 1997, 2nd edn, WHO, Geneva.
67. WHO. Strengthening Implementation of the Global Strategy for Dengue Fever/ Dengue Haemorrhagic Fever Prevention and Control. Report of the Informal Consultation. WHO/CDS/(DEN)/IC/2000.1. 2000, WHO, Geneva.
68. Gubler DJ. Dengue and dengue haemorrhagic fever. Clinical Microbiology Review , 1998, 11:480-496.
69. Kuno G. Review of factors modulating dengue transmission. Epidemiology Review, 1995, 17:321-335.

CHAPTER 7

Inequalities and Disparities in North Africa

Saber Boutayeb[1], Abdesslam Boutayeb[2,*] and Youssef Bensouda[1]

[1]*Institut National d'Oncologie Service Oncologie Médicale, Rabat, Morocco,*
Email: boutayebdr@yahoo.fr, Email: yoss.onco@hotmail.fr

[2]*Department of Mathematics Faculty of Sciences, Boulevard Mohamed VI, BP: 717 Oujda, Morocco*
Email: x.boutayeb@menara.ma

Abstract: Health and education constitute a cornerstone for human development of nations worldwide and especially for developing countries. In this context very few studies are devoted to Algeria, Egypt, Libya, Morocco and Tunisia as a group of countries forming what is called North Africa. These countries are often included in other regions like the Arab World, Africa, World Health Eastern Mediterranean Region (WHO-EMRO) and Middle East and North Africa (MENA). Belonging at the same time to Africa, Mediterranean Region, Arab World and Islamic countries, North African countries share language, religion and social and cultural custom. Consequently, it would be interesting to carry out a comparative study on their achievements in terms of human development and underlying components such as education, health, social welfare and violence.

Keywords: North Africa, education, health, equity, development, disparity, science.

1. INTRODUCTION

Health and education constitute a cornerstone for human development of nations worldwide and especially for developing countries. In this context very few studies are devoted to Algeria, Egypt, Libya, Morocco and Tunisia as a group of countries forming what is called North Africa. These countries are often included in other regions like the Arab World, Africa, World Health Eastern Mediterranean Region (WHO-EMRO) and Middle East and North Africa (MENA). Belonging at the same time to Africa, Mediterranean Region, Arab World and Islamic countries, North African countries share language, religion and social and cultural custom. Consequently, it would be interesting to carry out a comparative study on their achievements in terms of human development and underlying components such as education, health, social welfare and violence. Given that a large part of literature in North Africa is written in French and Arabic and hence not fully worldwide accessible, this humble contribution aims to summarize existing evidence in this region on the topic concerned. Globally, these countries are engaged in a multidimensional transition (demographic, economic, epidemiological and geographic) (Table **1**).

Table 1. North African countries: Demographic data as published by UNDP in 2008

	Algeria	Egypt	Libya	Morocco	Tunisia
Population(10^6)	32.9	72.8	5.9	30.5	10.1
% of Urban pop	63.3	42.4	84.8	58.7	65.3
% of pop under 15	29.6	33.3	30.3	30.3	26.0
% of pop aged 65+	4.5	4.8	3.8	5.2	6.3
GDP per capita PPP$	7062	4337	10335	4555	8371
Adult literacy (%)	69.9	71.4	84.2	52.3	74.3
Life expectancy	71.7	70.7	73.4	70.4	73.5
IMR (per 10^3)	34	28	18	36	20
MMR (per 10^5)	180	84	77	230	69

---

*Corresponding author

2. HUMAN DEVELOPMENT: SIMILIRATIES AND DISPARITIES BETWEEN COUNTRIES

We start by examining similarities and differences between North African countries according to the last available data on human development.

In North Africa, until recently, it was widely believed that economic development was a necessary prerequisite for improving a population's health status. But recent evidence showed that improved health is more than a consequence of development but rather a central axis of economic and social development. The introduction by the United Nations of human development index (HDI) as a mean of three indicators weighed equally: health (life expectancy at birth), standard of living (purchasing power parity income) and education (literacy and enrolment) illustrated clearly the importance of health and education and proved that an increase in national income alone does not capture development in its fullest sense [2,3]

As part of the Arab region, North African countries were concerned by the four Arab Human Development Reports. The first report (AHDR 2002)[4] diagnosed knowledge acquisition, freedom and good governance, and woman's empowerment as three cardinal deficits impeding human development in the Arab region in general. The second report (AHDR 2003)[5] was consequently devoted to education and knowledge acquisition, the third report (AHDR 2004)[6] dealt with freedom and governance, and finally a fourth report (AHDR 2005)[7] was dedicated to woman's empowerment. While noting the substantial economic and social progress made during the last decades, the previous reports stressed that Arab countries have accomplished less than expected in terms of human development globally and in education, health and social justice in particular.

The reports stimulated a controversial debate among Arab intellectuals and researchers.

Considering its resources, the Arab world has achieved less than expected in health and development according to some authors [8,9]. In another paper devoted to critical reflections on health and development in the Arab world, the author emphasized the need for consideration of social, economic and political issues in order to improve health and reduce poverty and inequalities [10]. The need to enhance education and consolidate democracy in the Arab world was also discussed [11,12]. Finally, in a paper dedicated to human development and health indicators in the Arab region [13], the authors carried out data analysis on education and health measures (omitting income), focusing on the link between human development and health indicators. Component Analysis was used to illustrate disparities and similarities among Arab countries. Although GDP *per capita* was not included in the analysis, the pattern illustrated by the first plan of Component Analysis (80% of information) was seen to agree fairly with the human development classification given by UNDP. Compared to oil-rich countries, North African countries were seen to have low rates of literacy and unacceptable low rates of access to health care and facilities, especially in rural areas.

Analysing the evolution of human development in North Africa, it appears that, during the last three decades, all countries had a similar increasing trend in human development index, although data is partly missing for Libya (Figure 1).

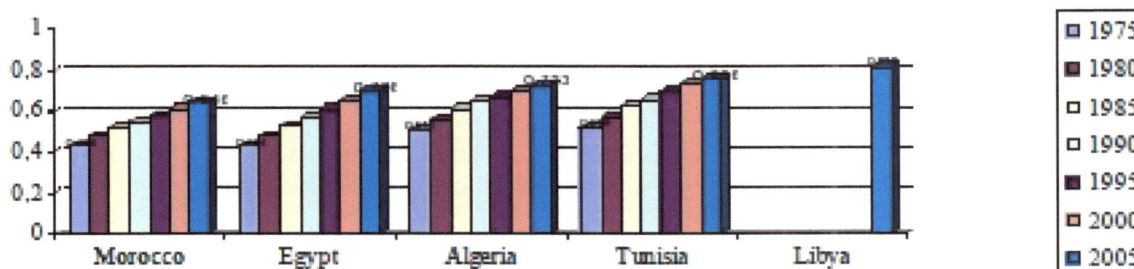

Figure 1. Evolution of human development index in North African countries.

Overall, Egypt achieved the best relative increase in human development index (63%) whereas Algeria had the lowest relative increase (43%). Morocco and Tunisia accomplished the same relative increase (48%). The Human Development Report 2007/2008[1] ranked Libya, Tunisia, Algeria, Egypt and Morocco respectively 56th, 91st, 104th, 112th and 126th amongst 177 countries worldwide. Accordingly, Libya belongs to the High Human

Development group whereas the remaining countries fall in the medium group. Libya and Morocco are separated by 70 countries, showing the gap existing between the two nations.

The human development index (HDI) being an average of three components, more details can be obtained by looking at the achievement of each country separately on health, education and income.

In 2005, all North African countries had a life expectancy at birth greater than 70 years (Table **1**). If we consider, however, the expectation of lost healthy years, these numbers will be amputated by 10 years or more.

In terms of education achievements, North African countries embarked upon the third millennium burdened by millions of illiterate adults (33%). For instance, in 2005 Morocco had nearly half of the adult population illiterate and less than 60% of combined gross enrolment in primary, secondary and tertiary education. Algeria, Egypt and Tunisia had adult literacy rates around 70% whereas Libya had a rate of 84.2%. Similarly, the rates of combined gross enrolment in primary, secondary and tertiary education where around 75% for Algeria, Egypt and Tunisia, and a higher rate for Libya (94.1%).

Looking at the between countries difference in income, it appears that GDP per capita in Tunisia ($8371) is nearly twice that in Morocco ($4555) and Egypt ($4337) and, although Algeria and Libya are both oil-countries producers, the Libyan GDP per capita ($10335) is much higher than GDP in Algeria ($7062).

As a conclusion, human development in North Africa is relatively uneven. As for life expectancy, the difference between Tunisia and Morocco is three years. In terms of adult literacy, the gap between Libya and Morocco is 32% and finally the Libyan GDP per capita is 2.4 times higher than GDP in Egypt.

3. INEQUALITIES AND INEQUITY WITHIN COUNTRIES

Human development index is among the most used indicator giving a summary measure of human development and allowing for comparison between countries around the world. However, although HDI deals with achievements in education, health and income in a given country, measurements are national average numbers which may hide inter-groups inequalities and regional disparities. Different forms of inequity remain not captured even with the use of measurements such as human poverty index (HPI), gender-related development index (GDI) and gender empowerment measure (GEM).

3.1 Measures of inequality

Consumption or income index is often used to measure economic inter-groups inequalities. For pragmatic reasons, however, wealth index is becoming the most used in research on economic disparities. This tendency is justified by the use of data collected through demographic health surveys (DHS) which contain no information on consumption and income but on the other hand, they do have sufficient data on assets necessary for a decent living standard and well-being (housing, access to water and sanitation, health services and health outcomes, education, employment, violence, leisure, etc...). Nevertheless, neither consumption/income nor wealth index is sufficient to define the multidimensional inter-group inequalities. Disparity and inequity can also be measured through education, gender, place of residence and other factors like ethnicity and stigma [14]. As explained by Marmot and Friel [15], evidence can be provided through analytical studies and/or randomised controlled trials.

Here, we rely on what is available for evidence in North Africa. Clearly, analytical analyses are used, based on data collected through publications in peer reviewed journals, reports released by international organisms such as the World Health Organization (WHO), the United Nations Children Fund (UNICEF), The United Nations Development Programme (UNDP), the United Nations Fund for Population (UNFPA), Population Reference Bureau, the World Bank and Social Watch reports; and national censuses and demographic health surveys (DHS).

3.2 Inequality in income or consumption in North Africa

Except the Libyan Arab Jamahiriya for which data is not available, with a slight gradient, the other countries have a similar pattern of income/consumption inequality. According to UNICEF and UNDP [1], in Morocco and Tunisia, the richest 20% absorb nearly 50% of all income/consumption, compared to 6.5 % or less for the poorest 20%. The ratio of richest 10% to poorest 10% reaches 13.4 in Tunisia (Mor:11.7, Alg: 9.6, Egy: 8) (Figure **2**). North African countries have a high Gini index compared to other countries (Alg: 35.3, Egy: 34.4, Mor: 39.5, Tun: 39.8). It is worth stressing that Tunisia which was seen to have better human development index than Algeria, Egypt and Morocco, is revealed as the country with the worst share of income/consumption. Globally, the four countries have unacceptable inequality in the share of income/consumption. This uneven distribution will certainly have consequences on the rates of poverty and access to basic social services like education and health but also on psycho-socio behaviours in general (violence, marginalization, mental illness, etc..).

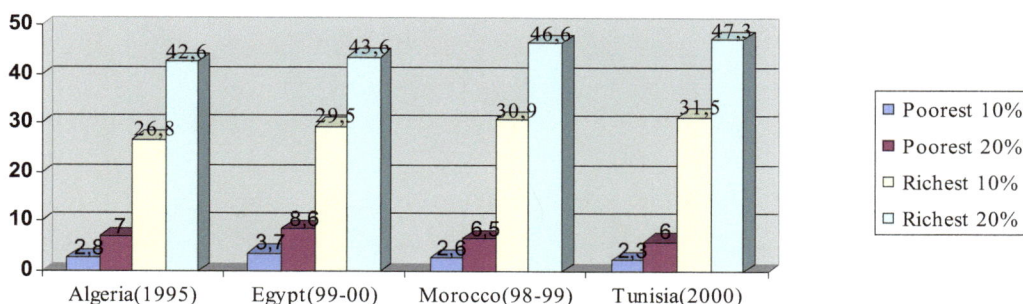

Figure 2. Inequality in the share of income or consumption.

3.3 Basic Capability Index (BCI)

Considering that poverty is a multi-dimensional phenomenon needing a conceptual framework based on the rights of persons (and not **on a markets**), Social Watch [16] has developed the Basic Capability Index (BCI) as a way to identify poverty not based on income but rather based on internationally development goals in terms of education, children's health and reproductive health. The BCI is based on three indicators: percentage of children reaching fifth grade, survival until the fifth year of age (based on mortality amongst children under five) and percentage of delivery assisted by skilled health personnel. Consequently, the highest possible BCI score is reached when all women receive medical assistance during labour, no child leaves school before completing the fifth grade and infant mortality is reduced to its lowest possible level of less than five deaths for every thousand. Accordingly, Morocco has a very low level (79), Egypt (88) is in the low level group, Algeria (94) and Tunisia (95) belong to the medium level class and Libya (98) is judged to have an acceptable level.

3.4 Children welfare and the Child Development Index (CDI)

Data on children's welfare is the most available. In its Report 2008, Save the Children indicates that across the world, 9.2 million children die every year before they reach their fifth birthday, 97% of all child deaths occur in 68 developing countries, one-quarter of all children worldwide are underweight, nearly one in three has stunted growth and 75 million primary school-age children are not enrolled in school, most of whom are girls. The report stresses further: "Outraged that millions of children are still denied proper healthcare, food, education and protection, we are determined to change this". The organization has consequently developed the Child Development Index (CDI) as a global multidimensional tool allowing to monitor how individual countries are performing in relation to the wellbeing of their children [17]. The proposed index is based on three components: under-five mortality, underweight and non-enrolment in primary school.

Figure (**4**) shows that North African countries achieved noticeable improvement in child well-being during the last fifteen years. Out of 137 countries for which data was available, Tunisia, Algeria, Egypt and Morocco are ranked 27th, 45th, 50th and 70th respectively. It should be stressed, however, that Morocco has accomplished the biggest improvement.

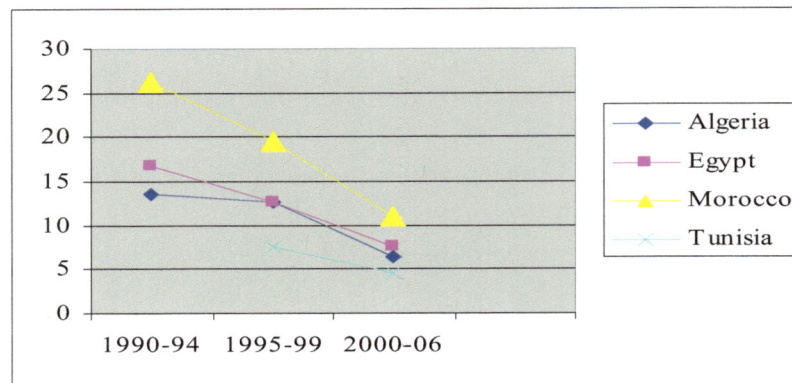

Figure 3. Evolution of Child Development Index in North Africa.

4. HEALTH EQUITY

Equity in health has become a central issue. However, equity can mean different things to different people. Moreover, the principles underlying its definition and conceptualization may vary with relation to economic, medical, philosophical, political, ethical and other considerations [18]. According to International Society of Equity in Health, equity in health is defined as the absence of potentially remediable, systematic differences in one or more aspects of health across socially, economically, demographically, or geographically defined population groups or subgroups [19]. Recalling that health was defined by the World Health Organization (WHO) as a state of complete physical, mental and social wellbeing and not merely the absence of disease or infirmity, the Alma Ata Declaration [20][42] stressed in 1978, that health is a fundamental human right and that the attainment of the highest possible level of health is a most important worldwide social goal whose realisation requires the action of many other social and economic sectors in addition to the health sector. Thirty years later, the WHO Commission on Social Determinants of Health[6] reaffirms the same statement in a more explicit form: "Where systematic differences in health are judged to be avoidable by reasonable action they are, quite simply, unfair. It is this that we label health inequity. Putting right theses inequalities -the huge and remediable differences in health between and within countries- is a matter of social justice. Reducing health inequities is an ethical imperative. Social injustice is killing people on grand scale". Advocating equity as a fundamental objective, the commission calls for a new approach to health and development. Action is recommended on three axes. First, improving the conditions of daily life in rural and urban areas, for men and women at all ages, focusing on early child development and adolescent, education and social protection. Second, addressing the inequitable distribution of power, money and resources, needing a strong public sector and better governance. And third, joining the efforts of professionals to those of civil society for action and assessment [21].

In the case of North African countries, health inequity can be illustrated on a multidimensional scale.

4.1 General pattern

Data from Demographic Health Surveys in Egypt, Morocco and Tunisia indicate that for health services like immunization coverage and contraception, inequalities are generally attenuated between rural and urban areas, rich and poor families, as well as between developed and deprived regions. This achievement is mainly due to national and international efforts based on generalised policies of public health with specified targets aiming to reach deprived and vulnerable populations. At the opposite side, other health services like antenatal visits, assisted births by skilled personnel and births given in health centres, as well as health outputs like infant and child mortality, stunting and underweight all show unjustifiable gaps between rural and urban; poor and rich; developed and deprived regions; and illiterate and educated women. Similar patterns are also found in access to basic services like drinking water and adequate sanitation.

4.2 Rural/urban and/or regional inequalities

In general all North African countries show rural/urban and/or regional discrepancies in health indicators and access to care. For instance, health indicators vary regionally between Lower Egypt and Upper Egypt, and, in each region, discrepancies are found between rural and urban populations [22]. Similarly, in Morocco, more than 30% of the rural population has to travel at least 10 kilometres to reach the nearest health facility, the number of inhabitants per physician ranges from 6362 in the rural area of Taounate (in the remote north east) to 380 in the capital, Rabat. The number of public hospital beds per 100 000 population ranges from 31 in the rural area of Berkane (in the remote north-east), to 444 in Rabat [9, 22].

The comparison between opportunities of access to health services in rural and urban populations in Egypt and Morocco indicates that the two countries have similar patterns of inequality between rural and urban populations (Figure **5**). A Moroccan rural woman is twice unlikely to attend antenatal care or to deliver with assistance of medical personnel; and nearly four times likely to deliver at home than a Moroccan urban woman. For Egyptian women, the ratios are respectively 0.5, 0.6 and 2.2. The low rates of access to essential maternal health services, with a great difference between rural and urban areas, may explain the high rates of maternal mortality and neonatal mortality [9, 22].

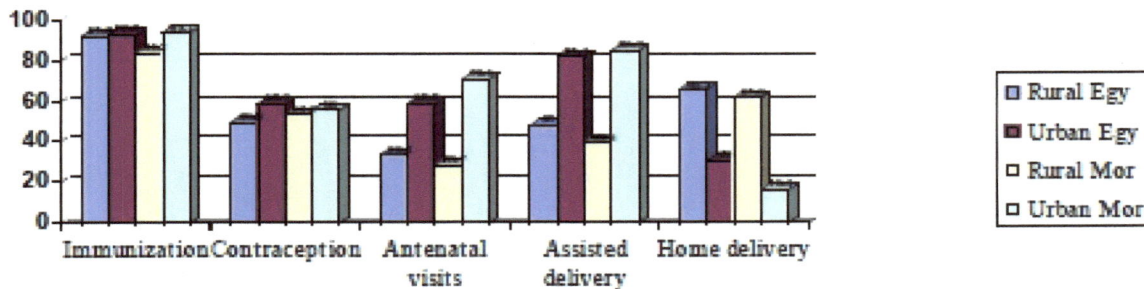

Figure 4. Rural-urban access to health services in Egypt and Morocco.

As for health outputs, Moroccan (respectively Egyptian) infant and children are twice (respectively one and half) likely to die or to suffer from stunting and under weight in rural areas than their counterparts in urban areas.

In Libya, effect of socioeconomic factors on child development were considered in a cross-sectional study carried out in two regions (Al Jabel and Tripoli) of the Jamahiriya on the growth and nutritional status of children under 5 years of age. The prevalence of stunting was higher among Al Jabel children (6.1%) than in Tripoli (2.5%) and in rural (6.8%) rather than urban (2.8%) areas [Jebal] [23].

4.3 Poor-Rich inequalities

Exacerbated inequalities are found in the use of health services such as antenatal visits, births assisted by skilled medical personnel and births given in a medical centre. In Egypt as in Morocco, the proportion of the richest women having multiple antenatal visits and that of women giving birth in presence of skilled personnel are threefold that of the poorest women. The gap in births given at home reaches fivefold in Egypt and twelve times in Morocco. As for health outputs, the pattern of inequalities in Egypt and Morocco are similar. The poorest children (respectively infant) are three time (respectively two and half) likely to die than the richest children and infant. Stunting and under weight reveal similar levels of inequality, with a fourfold gap in Moroccan underweight (17/4) (Figures **5.1** and **5.2**).

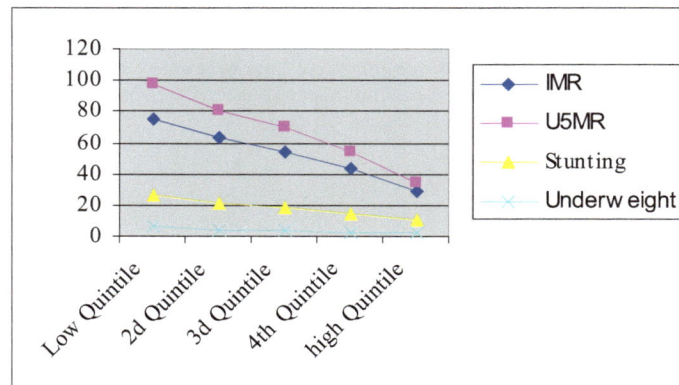

Figure 5.1: Health outputs in Egypt.

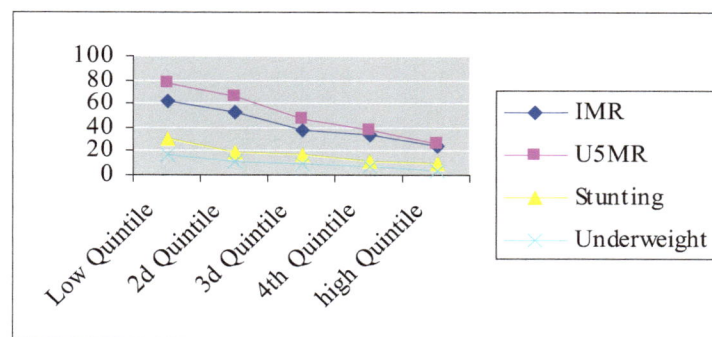

Figure 5.2: Health outputs in Morocco.

Two North African countries were amongst the 47 developing countries considered by Vand de Poel *et al* to analyse the relation between socioeconomic inequality and malnutrition in children aged up to 5 years. The authors used component analysis and a generalization of the concentration index, illustrating that socioeconomic inequality in malnutrition is present throughout the developing world [24].

In another study devoted to infant mortality in 16 Arab countries, socio-demographic, perinatal and economic factors were considered. Infant mortality was found to be inversely correlated to female and male literacy, GDP per capita, proportion of population with access to safe drinking water, and access to adequate sanitation facilities. Egypt, Morocco, Sudan, Yemen and Iraq were classified in the group with the highest infant mortality rate [25].

4.4 Health and Gender Equality Index (GEI)

Considering Gender Equality Index (GEI) based on empowerment, economic activity and education of women, the Social Watch report has shown that the score of North African countries is very low. Egypt, Morocco, Tunisia and Algeria scored respectively 40, 43, 49 and 52.

The same statement can be made by examining data provided by Demographic Health Surveys in Egypt, Morocco and Tunisia.

According to the author of a study in Islamic and Arabic countries, the low social and economic status of girls and women is a fundamental determinant of maternal mortality and reproductive health in many Islamic and Arab countries of which North African countries [26].

Using available data from national household surveys of 18 Arab countries, Khawaja *et al* analysed the impact of socioeconomic factors on child mortality and morbidity. Child health was measured by nutritional status, vaccination and Acute Respiratory Infection. Gender, residence (urban/rural), maternal education level, per capita GDP, female literacy rates, urban population and doctors per 100 000 inhabitants were used to describe and analyse within-country disparities in child health. The authors concluded that disparity by place of residence showed significantly higher rates of child mortality in rural areas and a similar trend in nutritional status. Whereas absence of gender disparity was noticed in immunization coverage. A noticeable disadvantage of illiterate mothers compared to mothers with at least secondary education was seen in wasting, stunting and vaccination rates [27].

5. EQUITY IN RESEARCH AND DEVELOPMENT: EXAMPLE OF CANCER

5.1 Introduction

Cancer is a leading cause of death worldwide in both developed and developing countries. In addition to heavy mortality due to cancer, there is a dual economic and psychosocial burden.

In the same way, one of the main objectives of health systems is equity. This concept refers to equality of opportunity and choice for all people, both within and between different countries.

The inequity is the result of disparities in incidence, diagnosis, treatment and mortality of cancer, but the major challenge in oncology is actually the burden of treatment especially chemotherapy and biotherapy.

Every year, several new molecules with high development coasts are approved for the cancer treatment.

All this news drugs are the fruit of the process of research-development in the industrialised world and is produced by the major pharmaceutical firms.

For the community, the burden of cancer care is growing exponentially making impossible the individual funding, so the intervention of health insurance organizations is mandatory.

But a major gap has widened between developed and developing countries due to the unequal resources. Populations from low-medium incomes countries have lot of difficulties to access to this new generation therapy. This inequality is reflected in ways downstream access to care asymmetric against cancer. Unequal intra and extra community is ultimately the result of a lack of a research / development in developing countries. This process involves a part of the epidemiology in each country, with the identification of priorities for research, a parallel investment in preclinical studies (drug discovery and animal testing) and Phase I, II and III results in obtaining permission to market the cancer drug. The loop continues as a share of profits related to the drug is returned to the research / development in order to perpetuate the process.

Until now, comparisons of data on cancer survival between high-income and low-income countries have not generally been available.

We suggest that international comparisons of cancer relative publications is very good indicator of the scientific performance on oncology.

Our aim is to prove that there is a strong relation between this " scientific performance" and the efficacy of the cancer health care system in each country.

We propose to evaluate the scientific global performance in oncology by the number of indexed article in Medline/Pub Med data base.

5.2 Example1: The inflammatory breast cancer

The inflammatory breast cancer (IBC) is the most aggressive type of localized breast cancer which have a specific epidemiology.

It represent about 1 to 2% of all breast cancer worldwide whereas is north Africa the rate of IBC is more than 6%.

As it was discussed before the asymmetric access to cancer treatment began by an insufficient epidemiological data then the deficit of basic research and clinical trials.

We propose in this article the number of articles listed in MEDLINE / Pub Med according the Keywords: inflammatory breast cancer + countries as an indicator of the performance concerning the "identification - solution" process (Table **2**).

Table 2. Scientific production concerning inflammatory breast cancer

Country	Number of articles in Medline	Country	Number of articles in Medline
Tunisia	8		
Morocco	0	USA	177
Algeria	0	France	56
Lybia	0	Italy	14
Egypt	3	**Global**	463
Lebanon	1		

Even if North Africa is considered worldwide as of high incidence area for IBC, only 11 from 463 listed on Medline for IBC was published in one of the north African (2.37%).

The analysis of these articles shows that 50% was published in collaboration with foreign scientists, at the opposite none of them was common between the north African countries.

The collaboration with the developed countries had a technical and financial value and makes easier the publication in the high impact factor journals.

5.3: Example2: Undifferentiated nasopharyngeal carcinoma

The undifferentiated nasopharyngeal carcinoma (UCNT) is a tumour of epithelial origin representing more than 90% of the nasopharyngeal carcinomas (NPC): cancers occurring in the nasopharynx, with particular epidemiologic characteristics. It is generally without any causal relation with tobacco or alcohol, but with multi-factorial aetiology implying genetic, environmental and viral factors, the EBV (Epstein Barr Virus) is frequently associated.

The geographical distribution of nasopharyngeal carcinoma (NPC) throughout the world is very particular, the incidence is variable, we distinguish areas of high incidence: in South-East Asia region, the disease is endemic, particularly in the South-East of China, the incidence occurs from 30 to 80/100 000/an. Intermediate rates are found in other regions of the South-East Asia, in North Africa, in the Middle-East region, and finally among the Eskimos of Alaska. Contrasting with these data, the incidence of the NPC is extremely rare, in Western Europe and in the United States (1/100000/year)

These particular epidemiologic data can be partially explained by the dietetic habits, the relationship to the consumption of meats and dried salted fish was shown in China accusing volatile nitrosamines like carcinogenic factors; in Tunisia, the exposure of spiced food containing "Harissa" since young age is blamed.

Table 3. Results of NPC study in Pub Med by countries

Country	Number of articles	Number of Study Phase II/III	Country	Number of articles	Number of Study Phase II/III
North Africa			**USA**	285	11
Tunisia	39	1			
Morocco	8	0	**Europe**		
			France	75	7
Algeria	2	0	Italy	33	4
Lybia	0	0	**South-East Asia**		
			China	1383	57
Middle East region			Indonesia	14	0
Sudan	1	0			
Egypt	4	1	Taiwan	361	13
Lebanon	1	0	Japan	130	9
Saudia Arabia	6	0	Malaysia	64	0
Turkey	48	2			

The NPC remain one of the serious public health problems in many countries in process of development, witch the disease is endemic (North Africa, South-East Asia). The lack of the epidemiologic and aethio-pathogenic data will do nothing but worsen the problem; indeed, the comprehension of the pathological mechanisms and the knowledge of the epidemiologic data specific to the country are essential to the improvement of the anti-tumoral therapeutic effect.

Our literature research reflects an important difference between the geographical distribution of the disease and the number of published studies; In fact we can distinguish three groups of countries:

The first group is particularly surprising, gathering many developed countries (France, United States, Italy), in witch the incidence of NPC is very weak, contrasting with the realization of several research and clinical studies. The population recruited often comes from the endemic zones, or are included in the oncologic centres of this countries by external scientific collaborators.

A second group comprises emerging countries, with high or intermediate incidence of NPC disease and logically has an important number of studies in Pub Med baseline, the republic of China is the first country regarding the published data, with an important impact in therapeutic management of NPC tumours in this country.

Lastly, the third group represented by countries in the process of development (North Africa, Egypt, Sudan, Indonesia), thus has a higher or intermediate incidence of NPC contrasting with the lack of scientific data, nevertheless more scientific activity is notable during the two last years; the alarming report still especially, in the negligible number of the phase II-III studies supposed to affect directly the diagnostic and therapeutic medical practices.

The difficulty of this third group of countries in producing research studies can be explained by several reasons: the absence of clinical research unit, the lack of medical ethic concept, there is also no formation for the medical and paramedical personnel. Also, as we seen, the majority of journal indexed are from developed countries, and they accept with difficulty, the articles or studies from poor countries. Finally the lack of resources and financial support for the realization of these research projects explain certainly this disappointing report.

Table 4. Results of cancer related articles in Medline/Pub Med by countries

Country	Number of articles in Medline	Country	Number of articles in Medline
Romania	1044	Poland	9130
Argentina	2772	Tunisia	680
Brazil	7612	Morocco	301
USA	457431	Algeria	114
France	49477	Egypt	1742
Italy	61028	Lebanon	67
Global	**2 273 470**		

5.4 Discussion

We also know that mortality information is essential for estimating relative cancer survival but sufficiently detailed mortality data are not available for the majority of developing areas, several countries are not covered by the cancer registries.

The first and the unique worldwide analysis of cancer survival, with standard quality-control procedures and identical analytic methods for all datasets is the concord study [28,29].

This study provides survival estimates for 1.9 million adults (aged 15-99 years) diagnosed with a first, primary, invasive cancer of the breast (women), colon, rectum, or prostate during 1990-94 and followed up to 1999, by use of individual tumour records from 101 population-based cancer registries in 31 countries on five continents.

Concord showed that Cancer survival varies widely between and within countries: the strongest indicator was the 5-year relative survival for breast, colorectal, and prostate cancer which was higher in North America, Australia, Japan, and northern, western, and southern Europe, and lower in Algeria, Brazil, and eastern Europe.

Inside the USA, the cancer survival was estimated in 11 countries covering 42% of the US population: Cancer survival in black men and women was systematically and substantially lower than in white men and women in all states included.

Moreover, inside Europe, two large studies Eurocare 3 and 4 showed a inter-country survival differences correlated to the rank on the total national expenditure on health (TNEH)[30,31].

The comparison between the data of Concord study and the table 3 which summarise the level of scientist production in the field of oncology proves that there is a correlation between the cancer survival and the index of scientific production.

Poverty contributes to an increase in cancer mortality and may be also incidence. The poorest communities have a higher incidence for several cancers and lower survival rates for all cancer sites combined [32-34].

A number of factors are truly responsible for the increased mortality and morbidity from cancer among the poor and include lack of employment, lack of education, inadequate housing, lack of access to medical care, chronic malnutrition, and a fatalistic attitude.

At the opposite in the developed countries a number of favourable factors are responsible for the decreased mortality and morbidity from cancer:

- ♦ Advances in the prevention.
- ♦ Early detection.
- ♦ Adequate treatment of cancer.

6. ACKNOWLEDGEMENTS

This paper was partly supported by a grant under the Global Project for Research (PGR) of the University Mohamed Premier, Oujda Morocco

7. DEDICATION

This humble contribution is dedicated to most disadvantaged people in North Africa

8. REFERENCES

1. UNDP. Human Development: Morocco 2007-2008. [http://hdrstats.undp.org/countries Accessed 30October 2008]
2. Boutayeb A. The double burden of communicable and non communicable diseases in developing countries. Trans. Royal Soc Trop Medicine and Hyg 2006; 99:191-199.
3. Marmot M, on behalf of the Commission on Social Determinants of Health. Achieving health equity: from root causes to fair outcomes. Lancet 2007; 370:1153-1163
4. UNDP. Arab Human development Report 2002. Creating Opportunities for Future Generations. [http://www.undp.org/rbas/ahdr/english2002.html Accessed 11 November 2005]
5. UNDP. Arab Human development Report 2003. Building a Knowledge Society. [http://www.undp.org/rbas/ahdr/english2003.html Accessed 11 November 2005]
6. UNDP. Arab Human development Report 2004. Towards Freedom in the Arab World. [http://www.undp.org/rbas/ahdr/english2004.html Accessed 11 November 2005]
7. UNDP. Arab Human development Report 2005. Woman Empowerment in the Arab World [http://www.undp.org/rbas/ahdr/english2005.html Accessed 1 February 2006].
8. Jabbour S. Health and Development in the Arab World: which way forward? BMJ 2003; 326:1141-1143.
9. Boutayeb A. Social Inequalities and health Equity in Morocco. Intern J Equ Health 2006. Available from http://www.equityhealthj.com/content/5/1/1
10. Jabbour S. Critical Reflections on Health and Development in the Arab World. Newsletter of the Economic Research Forum, for Arab countries, Iran & Turkey 2002; 9: 24-27
11. Fergani N. Second Arab Human Development Report : The need for a Knowledge Society. Newsletter of the Economic Research Forum, for Arab countries, Iran & Turkey 2003; 10: 10-11
12. Baroudi SE. The 2002 Arab Human Development Report: Implications for Democracy. Middle East Policy 2004; 11:132-140
13. Boutayeb A, Serghini M. Heath indicators and human development in the Arab region. Inter J Health Geogr 2006. Available from http://www.ij-healthgeographics.com/content/5/1/61
14. World Bank. Country report on Health, Nutrition and Population and poverty: Socioeconomic differences in health, nutrition and population.
15. Marmot M, Friel S. Global health equity: evidence for action on the social determinants of health. J Epidemiol ommunity Health 2008; 62:1095-1097
16 Social Watch. The Basic Capability Index. [www.socialwatch.org Accessed 2 December 2008].
17. Save the Children. The Child Development Index. London, The Save the Children Fund, 2008.
18. Macinko JA, Starfield B. Annotated Bibliography on Equity in Health, 1980-2001. Inter J Equ Health 2002. Available from http://www.equityhealthj.com/content/1/1/1
19. Starfield B. Improving equity in health: A research agenda. International Journal of Health Services 2001; 31(3):545-566
20.. Declaration of Alma-Ata. International Conference on Primary Health Care, Alma-Ata, USSR, 6-12 September, 1978 [http://www.who.int/hpr/NPH/docs/declaration_almaata.pdf]
21. Commission on Social Determinants of health. Closing the gap in a generation: health equity through action on the social determinants of health. Geneva: World Health Organization, 2008.
22. WHO. Building the knowledge base on the social determinants of health: Review of seven countries in the Eastern Mediterranean Region. Shoukrys CSDH evidence 7 counties. Geneva, World Health Organization, 2008, EMRO series 31.
23. Hameida J, Billot L, Deschamps JP. Growth of preschool children in the Libyan Arab Jamahiriya: regional and sociodemographic differences. East Mediterr Health J 2002; 8: 13-19

24   Vand de Poel E, Hosseinpoor A R, Speybroeck N, Ourti T V, Vega J. Socioeconomic inequality in malnutrition in developing countries. Bull World Health Organ 2008; 86(4), 282-91

25.   Shawky S. Infant mortality in Arab countries: sociodemographic, perinatal and economic factors. East Mediterr Health J 200; 7(6): 956-965

26   Kawaja M Dawns J Meyerson-Knox S Yamout R. Disparities in child health in the Arab region during the 1990s. Inter J Eq Health 2009. Available from http://www.equityhealthj.com/content/7/1/24

27.   Mohana N. Maternal Mortality in Islamic and Arabic Countries. Internet J Health 2005; 4:1

28.   Baili P, Micheli A, De Angelis R, Weir HK, Francisci S, Santaquilani M, Hakulinen T, Quaresmas M, Coleman MP; CONCORD Working Group. Life tables for world-wide comparison of relative survival for cancer (CONCORD study).Tumori. 2008 Sep-Oct;94(5):658-68

29.   Coleman MP, Quaresma M, Berrino F, Lutz JM, De Angelis R, Capocaccia R, Baili P, Rachet B, Gatta G, Hakulinen T, Micheli A, Sant M, Weir HK, Elwood JM, Tsukuma H, Koifman S, E Silva GA, Francisci S, Santaquilani M, Verdecchia A, Storm HH, Young JL; CONCORD Working Group. Cancer survival in five continents: a worldwide population-based study (CONCORD).Lancet Oncol. 2008 Aug;9(8):730-56. Epub 2008 Jul 17.

30.   Micheli A, Baili P, Quinn M, Mugno E, Capocaccia R, Grosclaude P; EUROCARE Working Group.Life expectancy and cancer survival in the EUROCARE-3 cancer registry areas. Ann Oncol. 2003;14 Suppl 5:v28-40. 31.   Mike Richards :EUROCARE-4 studies bring new data on cancer survival. *The Lancet Oncology, Volume 8, Issue 9, September 2007, Pages 752-753*

32.   Siminoff LA, Ross L. Access and equity to cancer care in the USA: a review and assessment. Postgrad Med J. 2005 Nov;81(961):674-9.

33.   Ward E, Halpern M, Schrag N, Cokkinides V, DeSantis C, Bandi P, Siegel R, Stewart A, Jemal A. Association of insurance with cancer care utilization and outcomes.CA Cancer J Clin. 2008 Jan-Feb;58(1):9-31. Epub 2007 Dec 20

34.   Wilkes G, Freeman H, Prout M. Cancer and poverty: breaking the cycle. Semin Oncol Nurs. 1994 May;10(2):79-88.

CHAPTER 8

Fifty Years of Human Development in Morocco: The Necessity of Equity Analysis

Abdesslam Boutayeb

[1]Department of Mathematics Faculty of Sciences, Boulevard Mohamed VI, BP: 717 Oujda, Morocco, Email: x.boutayeb@menara.ma

Abstract: Like many other developing countries, Morocco is struggling to achieve the main targets fixed by the Millennium Development Declaration for 2015. The report published in 2006 on *"Fifty years of human development in Morocco and perspectives 2025"* was a bold and praiseworthy initiative but it failed to carry out an equity analysis that indicates how to tackle the causes of the causes of persistent inequalities and disparities engendering underdevelopment. In this commentary, we give few examples illustrating the need to go beyond goals fixed in terms of average numbers, by tackling also the crucial problem of unfair and avoidable inequalities.

Keywords: Human development, equity, education, health, indicators, inequalities, disparities.

1. INTRODUCTION

In January 2006, the Moroccan authorities released a report entitled *"Fifty years of human development in Morocco and perspectives 2025"* [1]. The document was a synthesis of 75 individual contributions and 16 theme reports elaborated by a panel of experts. This praiseworthy initiative was qualified by the Regional Director of the United Nations Office for West Africa (UNOWA) as a good experience that should inspire African leaders and researchers to assess their fifty years of independence [2].

In April 2007, a conference on African human development was organized in Morocco, sponsored by the United Nations Development Programme (UNDP). Delegations from 47 African countries attended this meeting and adopted the Rabat Declaration, stipulating the promotion of solidarity between African countries and action for achievement of the Millennium Development Goals (MDGs). The declaration also encouraged the creation of an African network of experts in human development. The Second African Conference on Human Development is expected to be held in Gabon in 2009 [3]. While applauding the idea of the report assessing 50 years of human development in Morocco, and hoping that such an initiative will be followed by other African countries, we think that the report failed to give an equity analysis alongside assessment of human development achievements and/or Millennium Development Goals realizations. As stressed by the Commission on Social Determinants of Health, social justice is a matter of life or death [4,5]. Despite gains in average population health throughout the world, important disparities remain [6]. According to Gwatkin [7], government expenditures tend to benefit Africa's richest people more than its poorest in absolute terms. Although Morocco has achieved noticeable progress in terms of human development, important poor-rich and rural-urban gaps remain. Illustration is provided by the following examples [1,8].

2. REGIONAL DISPARITIES

During the last fifty years, the noticeable achievements accomplished globally in terms of human development were uneven and characterised by huge regional discrepancies. More than 30% of the rural population has to travel at least 10 kilometres to reach the nearest health facility, the number of inhabitants per physician ranges from 6362 in the rural area of Taounate (in the remote north east) to 380 in the capital, Rabat. The number of public hospital beds per 100 000 population ranges from 31 in the rural area of Berkane (in the remote north-east), to 444 in Rabat [9, 10]. Table1shows that, more generally, some regions are well developed and others marginalised. The highest HDI education component is twice that of the lowest region and the number of inhabitants per physician varies from 836 in the capital region to 4587 in the region of Taza-AlHoceima-Taounate.

Table 1. Huge disparities between regions

Region	HDI education	Inhabitants per physician	Inhabitants per dentist	HDI Global
Taza-AlHoceima-Taounate	0.337	4587	62034	0.541
Marrakech-Tensift-Al Haouz	0.394	3329	29404	0.565
Doukkala-Abda	0.405	3738	28909	0.566
Gharb-Chrarda-BeniHssen	0.426	2822	20871	0.574
Tadla-Azilal	0.427	4084	47200	0.577
Tanger-Tétouan	0.455	2611	21443	0.588
Souss-Massa-Draa	0.462	3539	32256	0.594
Oriental	0.480	2459	14646	0.598
Fès-Boulemane	0.486	2303	11321	0.598
Chaouia-Ouardigha	0.493	2750	27033	0.604
Meknès-Tafilalet	0.572	2729	23425	0.623
Guelmim-EsSemara	0.572	1918	104250	0.649
Rabat-Salé-Zemmour-Zaer	0.614	836	4769	0.660
Grand Casablanca	0.697	999	3870	0.697
Oued Ed-Dahab-Lagouira	0.739	1918	23000	0.740
Laâyoune-Boujdour-Sakia-El Hamra	0.768	1918	22444	0.742

3. RURAL/URBAN DIFFERENCES

Despite improvements in the global trend, many indicators show a persisting or even increasing gap between rural and urban areas. For instance, the ratio between the minimum salary in industry (SMIG) and its counterpart in agriculture (SMAG) has increased from 1·4 in 1960 to 1·5 in 2005. Similarly, the urban annual expenditure *per capita* in Moroccan dirhams (American dollars) has increased from MAD 5100 to 10600 (USD 607 to 1261) whereas in rural areas it has increased from MAD 3300 to 5300 (USD 393 to 631), indicating that in 2005 expenditure of urban populations is twice that of rural dwellers compared to 1.5 in 1960.

The comparison between opportunities of access to health services in rural and urban populations shows unacceptable differences (Figure **1**). A Moroccan rural woman is twice unlikely to attend antenatal care or to deliver with assistance of medical personnel; and nearly four times likely to deliver at home than a Moroccan urban woman. The low rates of access to essential maternal health services, with a great difference between rural and urban areas, may explain the high rates of maternal mortality and neonatal mortality [9, 10]. For instance, the average Moroccan level of maternal mortality is around three times that of Tunisia and 5.5 times that of Jordan (a country with a GDP per capita similar to that of Morocco)[10,11].

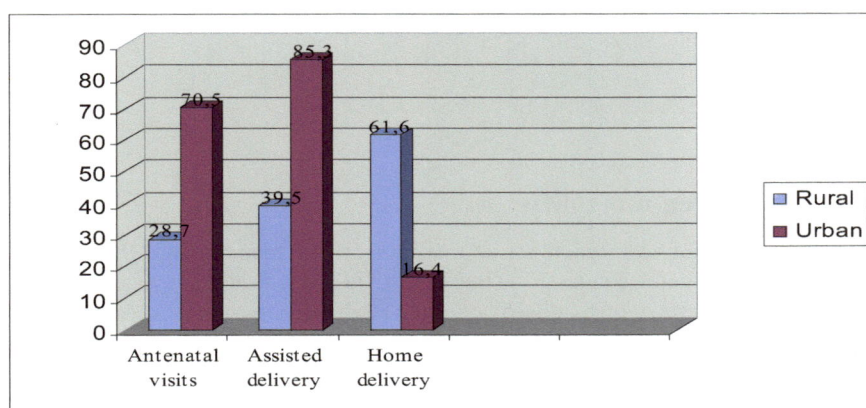

Figure 1. Rural-urban access to health services in Morocco.

4. POOR/RICH DIFFERENCES

4.1 Access to health facilities and health personnel

As stressed in the introduction, government expenditures tend to benefit Morocco's richest people more than its poorest in absolute terms. Inadmissible gaps exist in the use of health facilities and health personnel. Poorest women less likely to receive antenatal and/or postnatal care than richest women (Table **2**)[9-11].

Table 2. Access to health care facilities and health personnel

Socioeconomic Categories	Women who did not receive antenatal care (%)	Women who had no postnatal visit (%)	Women who gave birth at home (%)	Women who delivered with assistance of a traditional midwife (%)
Urban	15.1	83.7	16.4	7.7
Rural	52.1	96.4	61.1	33.8
R/U	3.5	1.2	3.7	4.4
Poorest quintile	60.3	97.1	70.5	39.9
Middle quintile	29.4	89.9	31.8	14.1
Richest quintile	6.9	73.6	6.0	3.1
Poorest/Richest	8.7	1.3	11.75	12.9

Another example is provided by the percentage of deliveries at home which has been reduced from 71·6% in 1992 to 38·5% in 2003. On average, the country has achieved important progress by nearly halving the percentage of women giving birth at home. Evolution is, however, uneven since the ratio between poorest and richest quintiles has increased from 3·3 to 11·8 in a decade or so. In terms of equity analysis, it is clear that the majority (94%) of richest women are using public and private centres for delivery whereas 70% of the poorest women are still delivering at home in unsafe conditions, exposing them (and their new born) to high risk of mortality and morbidity (Figure **2**).

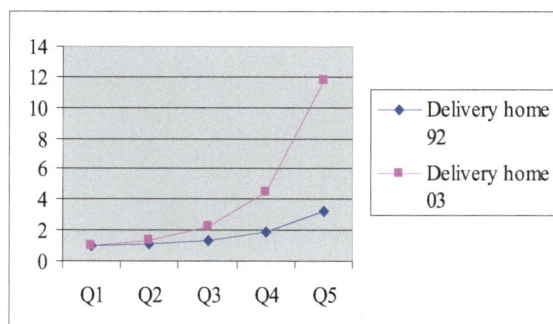

Figure 2. Delivery at home: evolution of the ratio poorest/richest.

4.2 Infant and Children mortality

Morocco is amongst the countries which are on track for achievement of the MDG4 (aiming to reduce by 2/3 the under five mortality rate in 2015 compared to the rate of 1990). Indeed, the mortality rate in children younger than 5 years (defined as the number of deaths of children under five years of age per 1,000 live births in a given population) has decreased from 89 in 1990 to 37 in 2006, and if the actual trend is maintained, Morocco will have reduced this rate by two- thirds, reaching 30 or less by 2015. However, if we consider the evolution of the same indicator in different socio-economic groups, we find that a poor child is threefold likely to die before his or her fifth birthday than a rich child. Moreover, the ratio gap has increased from 2·85 in 1992 to 2·98 in 2003 (Figure **3**).

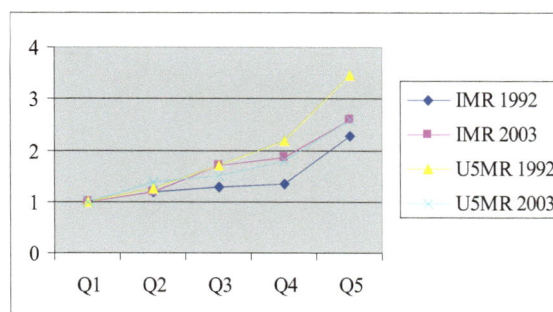

Figure 3. Infant and children mortality: evolution of the ratio poorest/richest.

5. ILLITERACY AND GENDER INEQUITY

One of the major problems affecting the human development index is the persisting rate of adult illiteracy. In fifty years, the adult illiteracy rate in Morocco decreased from 87% to 43% only. The report stressed the slow reduction by 1 to 2% per year but failed to give a comparison between rural and urban, men and women or between different socio-economic groups. In fact, the illiteracy ratio women/men has increased from 1·2 in 1960 to 1·8 in 2005, indicating that men benefited more than women from illiteracy reduction [10,11].

6. AKNOWLEDGEMENTS

This paper was partly supported by a grant under the Global Project for Research (PGR) of the University Mohamed Premier, Oujda Morocco

7. DEDICATION

This contribution is dedicated to the most disadvantaged populations in Morocco

8. REFERENCES

1. Royaume du Maroc. 50 ans de développement humain au Maroc et perspectives 2025.
    Accessible at http://hdr.undp.org/en/reports/nationalreports/arabstates/morocco/MOROCCO_2005_en.pdf
2. First African Conference on Human Development Declaration. Accessible at http://www.pnud.org.ma/pdf/DECLARATION.pdf
3. Le rapport (de l'ONU) sur le développement humain au Maroc. Accessible at http://www.droits-fondamentaux.prd.fr/codes/modules/articles/article.php?idElem=285613979
4. Marmot M., on behalf of the Commission on Social Determinants of Health. Achieving health equity: from root causes to fair outcomes. *Lancet* 2007; 370:1153–63
5. Commission on Social Determinants of health. Closing the gap in a generation: health equity through action on the social determinants of health. Geneva: World Health Organization, 2008.
6. Tugwell P, Petticrew M, Robinson V, Kristjansson E, Maxwell, L. Cochrane and Campbell Collaborations, and health equity. Lancet 2006; 367:1128–30.
7. Gwatkin D. The need for equity-oriented health sector reforms. Int J. Epidemiol. 2001; 30:720–23
8. Morocco Health Demographic Health Surveys. Accessed 03 October 2008
    http://www.measuredhs.com/countries/country_main.cfm?ctry_id=27
9. Boutayeb A. Social inequalities and health inequity in Morocco. Int J Equity Health 2005 doi:10.1186/1475-9276-5-1
10. WHO. Building the knowledge base on the social determinants of health: Review of seven countries in the Eastern Mediterranean Region. Geneva, World Health Organization, 2008, EMRO series 31.
11. Enquête sur la population de la santé familiale, Maroc, 2003-2004[PAPFAM]. Rabat, Ministère de la Santé , 2005.

CHAPTER 9

Children's Rights: A Multitude of Conventions and Declarations for a Miserable Situation

Abdesslam Boutayeb

Faculty of Sciences University Mohamed Ier, Oujda, Morocco,
Email: x.boutayeb@menara.ma

Abstract: During the last century, several international human rights conventions and political declarations have been adopted on children's rights alongside with regular reports released by organizations worldwide. The child rights were either stressed specifically or implicitly included as rights concerning all human beings. The spectre of children's rights is very wide, comprising, but not limited to, early development, education, health, recreation, physical, mental and spiritual development as well as protection against all kinds of exploitation, discrimination, cruelty and neglect. It is also constantly stressed that children should be entitled to these rights, without distinction or discrimination on account of race, colour, sex, language, religion, political or opinion. More attention is often devoted to children with specific needs like girls, orphans, disabled and those belonging to minorities or living in countries under war and conflicts. However, despite this arsenal of declarations and conventions, millions of children are still lacking the basic rights entitling them to a decent life with sufficient food, education, health facilities, dignity and other children's needs.

Keywords: Children, right, declaration, convention, health, education, wellbeing.

1. INTRODUCTION

During the last century, several international human rights conventions and political declarations have been adopted on children's rights alongside with regular reports released by organizations worldwide. The child rights were either stressed specifically or implicitly included as rights concerning all human beings. The spectre of children's rights is very wide, comprising, but not limited to, early development, education, health, recreation, physical, mental and spiritual development as well as protection against all kinds of exploitation, discrimination, cruelty and neglect. It is also constantly stressed that children should be entitled to these rights, without distinction or discrimination on account of race, colour, sex, language, religion, political or opinion. More attention is often devoted to children with specific needs like girls, orphans, disabled and those belonging to minorities or living in countries under war and conflicts. However, despite this arsenal of declarations and conventions, millions of children are still lacking the basic rights entitling them to a decent life with sufficient food, education, health facilities, dignity and other children's needs.

2. AN OVERVIEW OF DECLARATIONS AND CONVENTIONS ON THE RIGHT OF CHILDREN

2.1 Declaration of Geneva 1924

There is no doubt that children are amongst the most vulnerable groups affected by wars, conflicts and disasters. The necessity of aid and care for children who suffered from the consequences of World War I lead to the early creation of the Save Children International Union (SCIU) and consequently to the adoption of the Declaration of the Rights of the Child by the League of Nations in 1924. This Declaration, commonly known as 'Declaration of Geneva', calls for men and women of all nations, to give the Child the best that they can give, beyond and above all considerations of race, nationality or creed (See Box 1)[1]

Box 1: Geneva Declaration of the Rights of the Child (1924)

1. The child must be given the means requisite for its normal development, both materially and spiritually;
2. The child that is hungry must be fed; the child that is sick must be nursed; the child that is backward must be helped; the delinquent child must be reclaimed; and the orphan and the waif must be sheltered and succoured;

3. The child must be the first to receive relief in times of distress;
4. The child must be put in a position to earn a livelihood, and must be protected against every form of exploitation;
5. The child must be brought up in the consciousness that its talents must be devoted to the service of fellow men.

End Box 1

2.2 The Universal Declaration of Human Rights (1948)

Consequences of the World War II lead to the creation of the United Nations and other bodies like the World Health Organisation (WHO), the United Nations International Children's Emergency Fund (UNICEF) and others. One of the most known and cited declarations is the Universal Declaration of Human Rights adopted by the United Nations General Assembly in 1948. This declaration has dealt with the Child's rights implicitly and explicitly (Article25) (See Box 2)[2]

Box 2: Universal Declaration of Human Rights (1948)
> **Article1:** All human beings are born free and equal in dignity and rights. They are endowed with reason and conscience and should act towards one another in a sprit of brotherhood.
> **Article3:** Everyone has the right to life, liberty and security of person
> **Article25:** Motherhood and childhood are entitled to special care and assistance. All children, whether born in or out of wedlock, shall enjoy the same social protection.

End Box 2

2.3 Declaration of the Rights of the Child (1959)

Taking into account the Declaration of the Rights of the Child (1924), the Universal Declaration of Human Rights (1948) and statutes of other international organizations, The UN General Assembly proclaimed the Declaration of the Rights of the Child in 1959, aiming at a happy childhood and calling upon parents, upon men and women as individuals, and upon voluntary organizations, local authorities and national governments to recognize these rights and strive for their observance by legislative and other measures (See Box 3)[3]

Box 3: Declaration of the Right of the Child (1959)
> **Principle1:** The child shall enjoy all the rights set forth in this Declaration. Every child without any exception whatsoever, shall be entitled to these rights, without distinction or discrimination on account of race, colour, sex, language, religion, political or other opinion, national or social origin, property, birth or other status, whether of himself or of his family.
> **Principle2:** The child shall enjoy special protection, and shall be given opportunities and facilities, by law and by other means, to enable him to develop physically, mentally, morally, spiritually and socially in a healthy and normal manner and in conditions of freedom and dignity. In the enactment of laws for this purpose, the best interests of the child shall be the paramount consideration
> **Principle7:** The child is entitled to receive education, which shall be free and compulsory, at least in the elementary stages. He shall be given an education which will promote his general culture and enable him, on basis of equal opportunity, to develop his abilities, his individual judgement, and his sense of moral and social responsibility, and to become a useful member of society.
> **Principle8:** The child shall in all circumstances be among the first to receive protection and relief
> **Principle9:** The child shall be protected against all forms of neglect, cruelty and exploitation. He shall not be subject to traffic, in any form
> The child shall not be admitted to employment before an appropriate minimum age; he shall in no case be caused or permitted to engage in any occupation or employment which would prejudice his health or education, or interfere with his physical, mental or moral development.

End Box 3

Recalling the **inalienable** and indivisible rights proclaimed in the Universal Declaration of Human Rights (1948) and stressing that a child, by reason of his physical and mental immaturity, needs special safeguards and care, including appropriate legal protection, before as well as after birth, the UN General Assembly proclaimed the Declaration of the Right of the Child in 1959.

In 1989 the United Nations Convention on the Rights of the Child stressed responsibilities of society to protect children and provide them with appropriate support and services. It was further stated that children have the right to the highest attainable level of health and the right to a safe environment, free from injury and violence [4]. Children were also at the centre of the Resolutions WHA 56.24 on violence and health [5] and WHA 57.10 on road safety and health [6].

2.4 The World Conference on Human Rights: Vienna Declaration 1993

Fundamental human rights are posited as **inalienable** (individuals cannot lose these rights any more than they can cease being human beings); as **indivisible** (individuals cannot be denied a right because it is deemed a less important right or something non-essential); and as **interdependent** (all human rights are part of a complementary framework, the enjoyment of one right affecting and being affected by all others) [7]

Box 4: Vienna Declaration and programme of action (1948)

Article5: All human rights are universal, indivisible and interdependent and interrelated. The international community must treat human rights globally in a fair and equal manner, on the same footing, and with the same emphasis. While the significance of national and regional particularities and various historical, cultural and religious backgrounds must be borne in mind, it is the duty of States, regardless of their political, economic and cultural systems, to promote and protect all human rights and fundamental freedoms

Article18: The human rights of women and of the girl-child are an inalienable, integral and indivisible part of universal human rights. The full and equal participation of women in political, civil, economic, social and cultural life, at the national, regional and international levels, and the eradication of all forms of discrimination on grounds of sex are priority objectives of the international community

Article21: The World Conference on Human Rights, welcoming the early ratification of the Convention on the Rights of the Child by a large number of States and noting the recognition of the human rights of children in the World Declaration on the Survival, Protection and Development of Children and Plan of Action adopted by the World Summit for Children, urges universal ratification of the Convention by 1995 and its effective implementation by States parties through the adoption of all the necessary legislative, administrative and other measures and the allocation to the maximum extent of the available resources. In all actions concerning children, non-discrimination and the best interest of the child should be primary considerations and the views of the child given due weight. National and international mechanisms and programmes should be strengthened for the defence and protection of children, in particular, the girl-child, abandoned children, street children, economically and sexually exploited children, including through child pornography, child prostitution or sale of organs, children victims of diseases including acquired immunodeficiency syndrome, refugee and displaced children, children in detention, children in armed conflict, as well as children victims of famine and drought and other emergencies. International cooperation and solidarity should be promoted to support the implementation of the Convention and the rights of the child should be a priority in the United Nations system-wide action on human rights. The World Conference on Human Rights also stresses that the child for the full and harmonious development of his or her personality should grow up in a family environment which accordingly merits broader protection.

End Box 4

2.5 The Millennium Development Goals.

In 2000, the General Assembly of the United Nations adopted the Millennium Development Goals Declaration fixing eight goals to be reached by 2015. The first four goals are directly relevant to children in terms of nutrition, education and healthy survival. The remaining goals concern indirectly children. Moreover, it is stressed that "We will spare no effort to ensure that children and all civilian populations that suffer disproportionately the consequences of natural disasters, genocide, armed conflicts and other humanitarian emergencies are given every assistance and protection so that they can resume normal life as soon as possible"[8].

Table 1. The Millennium Project

Millennium Development Goals	Targets 2015
1. Eradicate extreme hunger and poverty	Reduce by half the proportion of people living on less than a dollar a day
2. Achieve universal primary education	Ensure that all boys and girls complete full course of primary schooling
3. Promote gender equality and empower women	Eliminate gender disparity in primary and secondary education preferably by 2005, and at all levels by 2015
4. Reduce child mortality	Reduce by two-third the mortality rate among children under five
5. Improve maternal health	Reduce by three quarters the maternal mortality ratio
6. Combat HIV/AIDS, malaria, and other diseases	Halt and begin to reverse the spread of HIV/AIDS. Halt and begin to reverse the incidence of malaria and other major diseases
7. Ensure environment sustainability	Reduce by half the proportion of people without sustainable access to safe drinking water Improve the lives of at least 100 million slum dwellers by 2020 Integrate the principles of sustainable development into country policies.
8. Develop a global partnership for development	

2.6 A world fit for children

In May 2002, a Special Session on children was held by the United Nations General Assembly. The output was a document "A world fit for children", aiming at a number of health goals for children, calling in particular, all Member States to "reduce child injuries due to accidents or other causes through the development and implementation of appropriate preventive measures"[9].

In the report released in 2008, the WHO Commission on Social Determinants of health indicated that populations' health is influenced by the conditions in which people are born, grow, live, work and age. In particular, child's environment influence his/her physical, emotional, mental and social development. The impact is so profound that it may affect health and wellbeing of a person during the whole life cycle [10].

The UNESCO Global Monitoring Report 2009 "Education for All" stresses that children in conflict-affected states are too often an absent constituency. In some cases, their lives are directly affected by violence and civil conflict. In others, their countries are undergoing post-conflict reconstruction [11].

3. THE CHILDREN'S SITUATION

3.1 Child mortality

Unfortunately, despite the arsenal of declarations and conventions adopted at different levels, millions of children are still lacking the basic rights entitling them to a decent life with sufficient food, education, health facilities, dignity and other children's needs. Although technological and medical progress have lead to noticeable achievements especially through vaccination programs and control of many childhood diseases, other diseases like AIDS, tuberculosis and malaria are still out of control in the majority of African countries. Children remain at high risk. Indeed, in 2002, of the 57 million deaths reported worldwide, 10.5 million deaths were among children of less than five years of age, of whom 98% were in developing countries in general and in Africa in particular. Deaths from underweight every year rob the world's poorest children of an estimated total of 130 million years of healthy life (Figure **1**)[12].

Rank	Cause	Numbers (000)	% of all deaths
1	Perinatal conditions	2 375	23.1
2	Lower respiratory infections	1 856	18.1
3	Diarrhoeal diseases	1 566	15.2
4	Malaria	1 098	10.7
5	Measles	551	5.4
6	Congenital anomalies	386	3.8
7	HIV/AIDS	370	3.6
8	Pertussis	301	2.9
9	Tetanus	185	1.8
10	Protein-energy malnutrition	138	1.3
	Other causes	1 437	14.0
	Total	10 263	100

(Reproduced by kind permission of the World Heath Organisation)

Figure 1. Child mortality in the six WHO regions, 2002.

3.2 The burden of HIV/AIDS

As stressed in the Millennium Development Goals, education is essential for human development and needs to be enhanced especially in low and medium income countries. Unfortunately, HIV/AIDS is reversing the trend towards the achievement of universal primary education in most African countries. In Africa, less than 65% of children are enrolled in primary school [13,14] and thousands of enrolled children will prematurely leave school under the pressure of HIV/AIDS including orphans, impoverished and those who withdraw to look after ill members of their families. In some African countries, nearly 50% of all orphans are due to AIDS (Table **2**). During the period 1999-2004, orphaned children represented 12.3% of all children under age 18 in Sub-Saharan Africa and the percentage of child labour reached 31.5%, 35.5% and 41% in Sub-Saharan Africa, Eastern and Southern Africa, and West and Central Africa respectively [15].

Table 2. Impact of orphan-hood on school attendance among 10-14 years-olds (%)

Percentage in school	West: 9 countries	Central: 6 countries	Eastern: 9 countries	Southern: 10 countries	All: 34 countries
Non-orphan	67	75	70	88	74
Orphan	58	69	54	84	69
Double orphan	57	58	49	80	64
Ratio double *vs.* non-orphan	.86	.94	.72	.90	.87

(Reproduced by kind permission of UNAIDS)

3.3 The WHO contrasting story

In the foreword to the WHO Report 2003, the WHO Director-General wrote:

"Two of the most striking findings in this report (WHO 2003) are to be found almost side by side. One is that in poor countries today there are 170 million underweight children, over three million of whom will die this year as a result. The other is that there are more than one billion adults worldwide who are overweight and at least 300 million who are clinically obese. Among these, about half a million people in North America and Western Europe combined will have died this year from obesity-related diseases…Could the contrast between the haves and have-nots ever be more starkly illustrated"[12]

3.4 UNICEF's devotion to children's cause

Since its establishment by the United Nations in 1946, UNICEF has spared no effort to help build a world where the rights of every child are realized. Many UNICEF's annual *State of the World's Children* reports have focused on specific issues such as nutrition, education, early development and HIV/AIDS.

In particular *the State of the World's Children* 2005 *"Childhood Under Threat"* offered an analysis of seven basic "deprivations" that children feel and that powerfully influence their future. The report indicated that: "More than one billion children are denied a healthy and protected uprising as promised by the 1989's Convention on The Rights of the Child (the world's most widely adopted human rights treaty). More than half the world's children are suffering extreme deprivations from poverty, war, and HIV/AIDS conditions that effectively deny children a **childhood** and hinder the development of nations. More than half the children in the developing world are severely deprived of one or more of the necessities essential to childhood (Table **3**).

Table 3. Seven basic deprivations

∞	640 million children do not have adequate shelter
∞	500 million children have no access to sanitation
∞	400 million children do not have access to safe water
∞	300 million children lack access to information
∞	270 million children have no access to health care services
∞	140 million children have never been to school
∞	90 million children are severely food-deprived

The UNICEF's State of the World's Children 2006

Under the title "Excluded and invisible", the UNICEF's State of the World's Children 2006 tackled the problems of millions of children who have not been the beneficiaries of past gains, the ones who are excluded or "invisible". According to this report, children are considered as excluded relative to other children if they are deemed at risk of missing out on an environment that protects them from violence, abuse and exploitation, or if they are unable to access essential services and goods in a way that threatens their ability to participate fully in society in the future. Children may be excluded by their family, the community, government, civil society, the media, the private sector and other children [16].

3.5 Save the children 2008 and the Child Development Index (CDI)

In its Report 2008, Save the Children indicates that across the world, 9.2 million children die every year before they reach their fifth birthday, 97% of all child deaths occur in 68 developing countries, one-quarter of all children worldwide are underweight, nearly one in three has stunted growth and 75 million primary school-age children are not enrolled in school, most of whom are girls [17].

Stressing that millions of children are still denied proper healthcare, food, education and protection, Save the Children has consequently developed the Child Development Index (CDI) as a global multidimensional tool allowing to monitor how individual countries are performing in relation to the wellbeing of their children. The proposed index is based on three components: under-five mortality, underweight and non-enrolment in primary school.

According to this indicator, North African countries have achieved noticeable improvement in child wellbeing during the last fifteen years. Out of 137 countries for which data was available, Tunisia, Algeria, Egypt and Morocco are ranked 27th, 45th, 50th and 70th respectively (Figure **4**). Analysing the impact of women's education on children's wellbeing, the Save the Children report stresses that: "Clearly, there is a strong relationship over time between women's empowerment and children's wellbeing; educated women are more likely to have healthy, spaced pregnancies, and subsequently healthy and educated children".

3.6 International Labour Organization (ILO) and child labour

According to International Labour Organization (ILO), some 352 million children between the ages of 5 and 17 were economically active worldwide in 2000, of which 246 million involved in what ILO defines as child labour which is to be eliminated [18].

In many developing countries, despite the existence of laws intended to protect children and prohibit their employment and abuse, boys and girls are exposed to child labour, sexual tourism and different forms of exploitation and neglect.

3.7 Social Watch Report and Basic Capability Index (BCI)

Stressing the growing phenomenon of street children, the last Social Watch Report estimates

Considering that poverty is a multi-dimensional phenomenon needing a conceptual framework based on the rights of persons(and not on a markets), Social Watch has developed the Basic Capability Index as a way to identify poverty not based on income but rather based on internationally development goals in terms of education, children's health and reproductive health. The BCI is based on three indicators: percentage of children reaching fifth grade, survival until the fifth year of age and percentage of delivery assisted by skilled health personnel. Consequently, the highest possible BCI score is reached when all women receive medical assistance during labour, no child leaves school before completing the fifth grade and infant mortality is reduced to its lowest possible level of less than five deaths for every thousand. Worldwide, countries are classified according to the level of this index (very low, low, medium, and acceptable level) [19].

4. THE GAZA'S CHILDREN CASE STUDY

4.1 Consequences of occupation on children

Since the invasion by Israel in 1967, occupation, deprivation, restriction of movement and frustration from a secure decent life had a devastating effect on the psychological behaviour of men, women and children. The whole population is feeling a permanent imprisonment. In face of Israeli soldiers armoured with sophisticated weapons, constantly provoking, abusing and violating all human rights, Palestinian children have come to throw stones as a last resort to express their rejection of occupation and the need for a flourishing life like all children of the world.

Although the Israeli response to the first uprising (Intifada) (1989-1993) was lethal, it hardly compares to the more violent response to the second uprising which started in 2000. It is estimated that about one thousand children were killed between October 2000 and 25th December 2008, before the launch of the Israeli attack in 27th December 2008. Under Israeli occupation, however, death numbers give only a partial picture of the suffering incurred by the Palestinian population in general and children in particular. According to a Queen's University study in 2006, most children in the Gaza Strip have been tear gassed, have had their homes searched and damaged, and have witnessed shooting, fighting and explosions. Many have been injured or tortured as a result of chronic war that spans generations. Consequently, 98% of Gaza's children do experience or witness war trauma. The study indicates that a child who had a severe head injury has 4 times the risk of emotional disorder. A child who has witnessed friends injured or killed has 13 times the risk of Post Traumatic Stress Disorder [20].

Since the second Intifada in 2000, the humanitarian situation has been deteriorating as a consequence of successive blockades imposed by Israel on Gaza strip.

In February 2008 UNICEF wrote that "Children make up more than half of the 1.4 million residents of the Gaza Strip in the Occupied Palestinian Territories. Gaza's children, inheritors of the world's longest-running conflict, now also bear the brunt of new import and border controls" [21].

In a report published in Mars 2008, a group of eight humanitarian organizations based in UK, affirmed that Gaza strip was facing the worst humanitarian crisis since the occupation by Israel in 1967. The impact was particularly felt in health conditions and children were amongst the most vulnerable people [22].

In 30th April 2008, the UNRWA director judged that Gaza's population was in a shocking and shameful situation.

4.2 Children under Israeli war

As expressed by the EMRO-CSDH, conflict and its consequences destroy health and infrastructure, and cause death and destruction, loss of human rights and widespread of mental health problems[23].

This is exactly what happened when Israel launched its attack against Gaza strip in 27th December 2008.

During three weeks of a devastating war on the densely populated city of Gaza, the Israeli army has killed nearly 1350 people (of whom more than 400 children and 100 women) and injured some 2000 children among a total of 5500 people injured. But the consequences of the destructive attack on Gaza's children are still to come. Indeed, those who escaped from death and physical injury will have to endure the prolonged emotional effect of war. The quasi-totality of the 800 000 Gaza's children have witnessed the killing and massacre of their family members, friends or neighbours. They have seen destruction, demolition and shelling of their home, schools, health centres and even UNRWA's warehouse facilities and workshops which provide aid to 70% of Gaza's population. Forty five children were killed by a single shell on one of the schools used by UNRWA as a shelter for children and families who left their home under Israeli attack.

The World Health Organization expressed concern about management of chronic disease patients and public health in Gaza Strip. The child vaccination programme and the surveillance of water quality were seriously affected, which may result in epidemics in a city, where the existing risk due to a high population density living in dire conditions, is now augmented by the consequences of war [24].

The UN General Secretary qualified the Israeli attack on schools operated by UNRWA as totally unacceptable since the Israeli authorities were informed and knew that these schools were under the supervision of United Nations. He also affirmed that the number of people killed by the Israeli army reached an unbearable point.

The UNICEF reiterated several times its call for the end of violence, stressing that children in Gaza are currently deprived not only of the basic human rights any human being should enjoy but are also denied the fundamental rights specific to children such as the right to be protected from all forms of physical or mental violence and injury, and the right to education, development and access to healthcare services [21].

A multitude of other voices were raised to denounce the barbarism of Israeli army on children, women and civilian in general. Worldwide, people were struck by the savage attack on civil infrastructure, demolishing schools, hospitals, mosques and other services.

For Gaza's children, however, the massacre seemed to be just contemplated by the whole world, unable to respond to their repetitive call under fire and stress caused by a sophisticated army using all kind of weapons, including phosphorous bombs and other internationally prohibited weapons.

The World Health Organization estimates that between 70% and 75% of a population develop mild to moderate post-traumatic reactions after a large-scale crisis such as the one in Gaza, while it estimates that 5% to 10% of people in Gaza may need professional mental health support to address more long-term problems, such as depression, trauma, anxiety, and panic attacks[25].

5. ACKNOWLEDGEMENTS

This paper was partly supported by a grant under the Global Project for Research (PGR) of the University Mohamed Premier , Oujda Morocco

6. DEDICATION

This contribution is dedicated to Gaza's children

7. COMPETING INTERESTS

I declare that I have no competing interest

7. REFERENCES

1.   United Nations. Universal Declaration of Human Rights. Geneva. 1948
      [http://www.un.org/Overview/rights.html accessed 1 April 2009]
2.   Geneva Declaration on the Rights of the Child 1924
      [http://www.un-documents.net/gdrc**1924**.htm accessed 2 April 2009]
3.   United Nations Declaration of the Right of the Child 1959
      [http://www.unhchr.ch/html/menu3/b/25.htm accessed 28 April 2009]
4.   UN. Convention on the Rights of the Child. New York, NY,United Nations, 1989.
5.   WHO. Implementing the recommendations of the World report on violence. Geneva, World Health Organization, 2003, Resolution WHA56.24
6.   WHO. Road safety and health. Geneva, World Health Organization, 2004, Resolution WHA 57.10
7.   United Nation Vienna Declaration and Programme of Action 1993
      [http://www2.ohchr.org/english/law/pdf/vienna.pdf accessed 25 April 2009]
8.   UN. United Nations Millennium Declaration. New York, NY, United Nations, 2000
9.   UN. A world fit for children. New York, NY, United Nations General Assembly, 2002.

10. Commission on Social Determinants of health. Closing the gap in a generation: health equity through action on the social determinants of health. Geneva: World Health Organization, 2008.
11. UNESCO. Education foe All Global Monitoring Report 2009 Oxford University Press, 2009
12. WHO. The World Health Report 2003: Shaping the Future. World Health Organization Geneva, 2003a.
13. UNESCO: Education for All in Least Developed Countries. [http://unesdoc.unesco.org/ accessed 15/10/2007]
14. UNICEF: The state of the world's children 2006. The United Nations Children's Fund, 2005.
15. Boutayeb A. The Impact of HIV/AIDS on Human Development in African Countries.
16. UNICEF: The state of the world's children: Excluded and Invisible. New York: The United Nations Children's Fund 2006
17. Save the Children. The Child Development Index. London, The Save the Children Fund, 2008.
18. International Labour Organization. [http://www.ilo.org Accessed 10 October 2008]
19. Social Watch. The Basic Capability Index. [www.socialwatch.org Accessed 2 December 2008]
20. SienceDaily. Ninety-eight Percent of Gaza's children experience or witness war trauma. [http://www.sciencedaily.com/releases/2006/08/060801183448.htm accessed 12 January 2009]
21. UNICEF: [http://www.unicef.com]
22. Amnistie Internationale, CARE International UK, CAFOD, Christian Aid, World Physicians, UK, Oxfam, Save the Children UK and Trocaire. The Gaza Strip: A Humanitarian Implosion. London, UK, 2008.
23. WHO-EMRO. Building the knowledge base on the social determinants of health. WHO Regional Publications, Eastern Mediterranean Series 31, 2008
24. WHO [http://who.int.org Accessed 10 December 2009]
25. Gavlak D, Jamjoum L. Rebuilding lives, healing minds. Bull World Health Organ 2009; 87:408-409.

Subject index